THE SCANDINAVIAN BELLY FAT PROGRAM

Berit Nordstrand

THE SCANDINAVIAN BELLY FAT PROGRAM

12 weeks to get healthy, boost your energy and lose weight

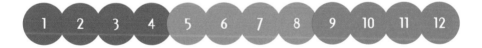

Berit Nordstrand

Photography: Studio Dreyer Hensley

MURDOCH BOOKS
SYDNEY · LONDON

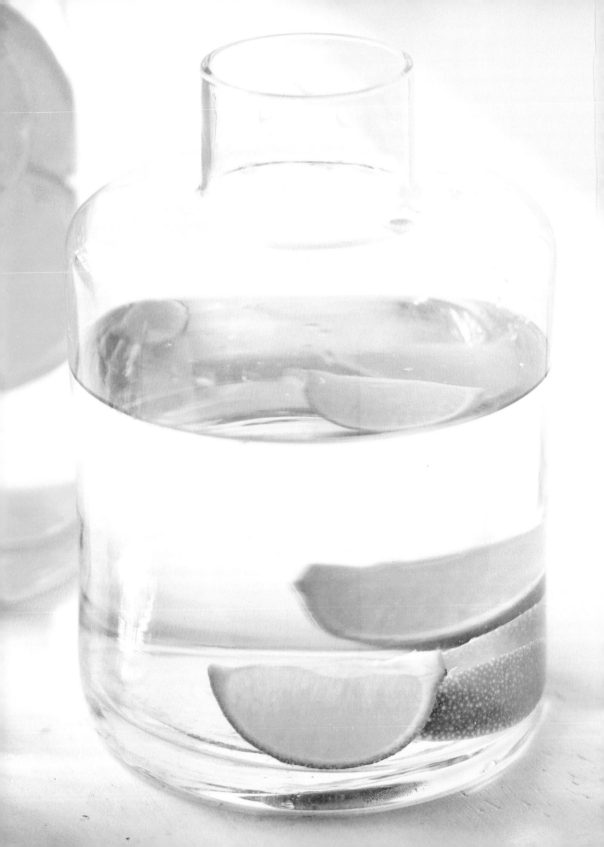

CONTENTS

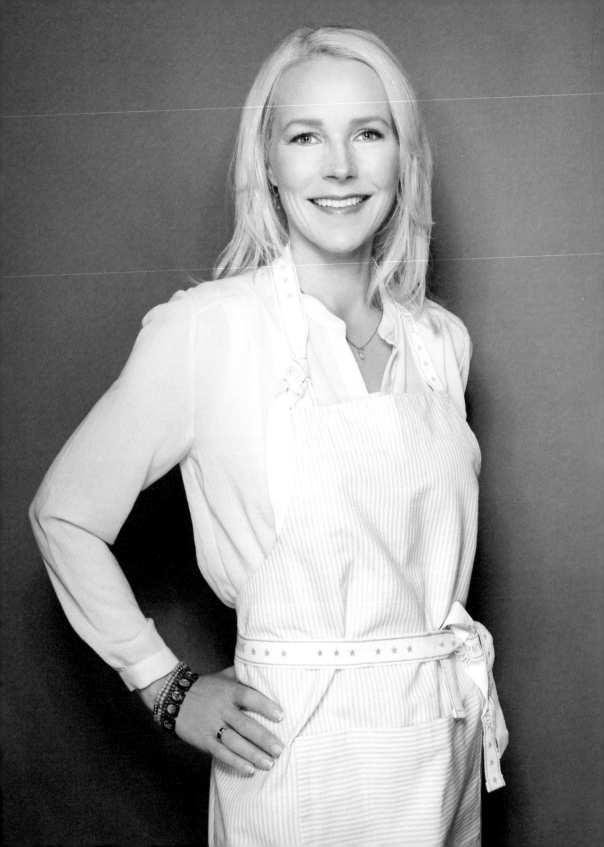

INTRODUCTION

If you are like most people, you will have fought against excess weight on numerous occasions, but lost hope due to demanding diets and training schedules. Maybe you have repeatedly struggled *against* your body and starved yourself for long periods of time, only for the kilos to pile on again, and to find that the suffering was all in vain. Did you step back, discouraged, with the feeling that you lack willpower, and did you give up the goal of an energetic, happy and slimmer body? Don't lose faith. I'm pretty sure you've fought a battle *against* yourself – a battle that is impossible to win! Now is the time to replace that struggle with enjoyment. Yes, you read that right. Here you will be given a simple initiation on how to live with your body – and how to combine both a reduction in your weight, and a slimmer waist, with more enjoyment over the course of your hectic daily life. By living more in tune with your body's needs and natural rhythms, and by selecting ingredients that keep the fat burning, gradually you will achieve a flatter stomach and win the battle against excess weight for good.

It was during a difficult period of my life that I discovered the need to top up my positive energy and brainpower, because I was constantly drained of both strength and courage. I found that my batteries were recharged through the senses and mindfulness, by pleasure rather than by struggle. Furthermore, numerous experiences with patients (addicts who have found their own key to lasting change) convinced me that there are several approaches that would work for most of us – clear short-term objectives, a focus on mastery of the goal, methodical observation, and more joy. For me, a treat might be an extra special evening meal, a barbecue on the beach, a boat ride, meeting friends or indulging in a spa in my own bathtub. You charge your batteries and live more harmoniously with your body's needs when you engage in activities that you know give *you* pleasure.

More and more of us struggle with excess weight that reduces our quality of life. Although the body cannot do without fat to keep us warm and as a source of energy in bad times, too much fat translates into health problems. It's important to note that very few of us experience those bad times, so our stores of fat are loaded up but never used. In 2010 the World Health Organization estimated that more than 40 million, or 6.7%, of the world's children under five were overweight (de Onis 2010). There is a lack of recent data for Australia, but a study done in 1995 showed that 20–21% of Australian children aged between seven and 15 years were considered to be overweight or obese (Magarey et al 2001). These figures show a tripling of the prevalence of obesity in the ten years from 1985. In New Zealand, a survey done in 2014–15 revealed one in nine children (aged 2–14 years; 11%) were obese (NZ Ministry of Health 2015). If you are overweight as a child, the risk of health problems, obesity and premature death as an adult increases substantially. In 2004–05 in Australia, 41% of males and 25% of females were classified as overweight, and 18% of males and 17% of females were classified as obese (Australian Bureau of Statistics 2005). With obesity comes an increased risk of type-2 diabetes, inflammatory ailments, pain, cardiovascular disease and various types of cancer. Health problems such as abdominal pain, headaches, diminished concentration, impaired memory, restless sleep, anxiety and/or depression can result. Too much fat around the waist causes more general physical problems than you might imagine.

Previously it was thought that extra fat on the body was just an unnecessary load, and that it could be compared to carrying around a backpack. Now we know that while fat around the hips and buttocks remains steady, and can be compared to the fat along the edge of a pork chop, there is a lot of activity in the abdominal fat cells. Excess abdominal fat cells are like small chemical factories that produce harmful inflammatory substances. Here fat cells are depleted and replenished all the time, and the blood continuously seeks nourishment from the fat cells in the belly so that you can be nourished in the 'fasting part' of the day – in other words, while you are sleeping. We need a little belly fat, but nowhere near the quantities many of us have today.

If you have several kilos of excess fat, it needs oxygen and nutrients. It means that your heart has to work hard to pump blood through mile after mile of narrow veins in the abdominal fat cells. It's a bit like trying to blow up a tiny balloon – you really have to blow hard to fill it with air. In the same way, the heart muscle pumps heavily in order to push blood into the arteries at a suitable pressure to reach the many kilos of unnecessary fat. Then your blood pressure will usually rise. In individuals with genetic risk factors, blood pressure will rise rapidly.

In the fat cells, inflammatory substances called cytokines are produced that can lead to water retention, swelling and body pain. The inflammatory substances also graze the walls of the arteries from the inside, so cholesterol and fats in the bloodstream can easily establish themselves. In addition, the inflammatory substances numb the cells' receptors so that sensitivity to hormones and neurotransmitters is impaired. Because of this you experience lower levels of happiness and motivation from dopamine and norepinephrine, and a reduced sensation of satisfaction from the fullness hormones. Insulin, the blood sugar or glucose regulator, no longer acts effectively. The body's ability to control blood sugar is extremely important, so the body will quickly try to compensate for the effect of weakened insulin and the fact that the cells do not absorb glucose as easily. It does this by increasing insulin production. With a few additional kilos of belly fat and a waist measurement of more than 80 cm (31½ inches) for women and 94 cm (37 inches) for men, the chemistry in the fat cells drowns the insulin hormone's messages to them. This causes 'impaired insulin detection', or what is called insulin resistance. If the belly fat cells continue to dominate, you will eventually develop type-2 diabetes.

Belly fat is the scariest fat you have on your body! Belly fat causes problems in multiple organ systems and is a contributing cause of cardiovascular diseases, asthma, migraines, rheumatism and cancer. When the inflammatory reaction reduces sensitivity to serotonin, dopamine and norepinephrine – neurotransmitters in the brain that control pleasure and motivation – you feel depressed. We are not talking about a backpack that is just a burden to carry around, but something far more serious. So it's wonderful for you and your health that you have started reading this book. You will be introduced to a method and a way of life that delivers more pleasure, a better quality of life, a lighter body and a brighter mind.

MEN: WAIST MEASUREMENT > 94 CM (37 INCHES) = OVERWEIGHT
WAIST MEASUREMENT > 102 CM (40⅙ INCHES) = OBESE
WOMEN: WAIST MEASUREMENT > 80 CM (31½ INCHES) = OVERWEIGHT
WAIST MEASUREMENT > 88 CM (34⅔ INCHES) = OBESE

It is not your body weight in itself that curbs your energy – it is the aggressive abdominal fat cells that work against you. One of my patients was 1.7 m (5 ft 7 inches) tall and weighed 65 kg (143 lb 5 oz). She wasn't overweight – she didn't have a body mass index (BMI) over 25 – but suffered from low energy, depression, anxiety and declining concentration. Through guidance and supportive chats she changed her eating habits and began to go for evening walks. Over the course of a few weeks she lost several kilos of fat around the waist, and her mood, concentration and vigour improved. She was shocked by how a little extra on the belly can spoil life's pleasures. Even if you have an acceptable BMI, the abdominal fat cells create bigger problems for you than just your jackets being a little too tight around the waist. If, slowly but surely, the kilos have sneaked up on you again, now they will gradually disappear, while you focus on moving a little more, getting enough sleep, relaxation, pleasure, and the great taste of real food.

With a few simple steps, you are going to learn how you can focus on more everyday pleasure – with the wonderful result that the body shifts over into fat-burning mode, so that the belly fat steadily disappears. Then you can forget about counting the calories and constantly fighting hunger, because total body weight is about much more than a simple accounting for energy – or calories in and calories out. It is about an imbalance on your plate, a lack of necessary nutrients, about stress, instability in the stomach, quiet inflammation, and the unfulfilled need for comfort. While some foods settle as fat around the waist, others are capable of increasing the burning of fat. Calories from refined white carbohydrates, especially, are stored as fat around the waist. I'll come back to this shortly.

In this book you will get simple tips and tricks, spread over 12 weeks, which will help you to speed up the burning of fat, increase muscle mass, reposition fat around your body, and reach your ideal waist size.

Moving a little more and increasing your energy consumption will contribute to real weight loss, not just a transfer of the harmful belly fat to the hips and the bottom. Reduced daily 'chair time', some evening walks and simple strengthening exercises at home show fantastic results. Gradually you may also get motivated to spend a few hours at the gym. Weigh yourself once a week, but be patient on the scales. Remember that muscle weighs more than fat, so replacing fat with muscle mass does not necessarily make much impact on the scales in the first few weeks. If you are overweight, a reduction in weight of 5% mainly targets dangerous abdominal fat, and you will achieve great benefits for health, as well as a body weight and a waist size that you can be happy with.

It is more important for your health to reduce waist size than to reduce weight. Get rid of the belly fat that unleashes all kinds of chemicals and limits your quality of life. Shut down the fat cells, stop them reproducing, and experience a significant and lasting improvement in your quality of life.

YOUR WAISTLINE IS YOUR LIFE LINE – LET'S GET STARTED!

PREPARATIONS TO HELP YOU REACH YOUR GOALS

It is easier to start a good habit than to stop a bad one. Here you'll learn how to get going.

1   If your dinner plates are enormous, buy some slightly smaller ones. Since the eyes are bigger than the stomach, a fuller small plate feels more satisfying than a half-filled huge one.

2   It is easier for you to practise portion control, or to eat until you are full, if you eat slowly. This gives the fullness hormones time to make you feel satisfied before you eat too much. Decide to eat until you are 'not hungry' instead of 'very full'. This will shrink the size of your stomach a little, so that eventually you will feel full even if you eat a little less.

3   Buy different kinds of green tea and enjoy a cup before, during and after mealtimes. Taking a warm drink will slow down your eating in a natural way. (Are you in a rush? Then move the meal to another time!)

4   Stabilise blood sugar and reduce cravings by eating little and often. Get hold of an old chalkboard and hang it on the kitchen wall. It's decorative! Write down the time of the main meals until they are established as new daily routines.

5   Remember that 'drowsy' does not mean 'hungry', even though you crave an energising snack because the brain thinks that your blood sugar is too low. It is *protein* that you are missing, not sugar, when you feel those cravings.

6   Teach yourself to understand how hungry you are before you eat. On a scale from 1 (extremely hungry) to 10 (extremely full), how hungry are you really? At 5 you are no longer hungry, and at 6 you are satisfied. Spend some time considering if you really are still hungry before you fill your plate again. With regular eating times, it is never long before your next meal that you'll need room for!

7   Always drink a glass of water or a cup of tea before meals. This will significantly increase weight loss throughout the 12 weeks you have ahead of you.

8   Enjoy yourself more! Chew a little longer on every mouthful that you take and savour the tastes of the pure ingredients. Then you will experience more pleasure and fewer cravings.

Helpful tips for when you have cravings

NOW YOU WON'T HAVE TO LOSE THE BATTLE AGAINST THE CRAVINGS THAT TORMENT YOU – YOU CAN LEARN HOW TO TAKE CONTROL OF YOUR APPETITE.

1. Eat a little every 3–4 hours.

2. Choose snacks wisely. Smart snacks between main mealtimes keep the blood sugar stable and sugar cravings at a distance, while increasing the metabolism.

3. Make a plan in advance so that you know what to do when the cravings creep up on you. Regardless of whether the cause of the cravings is habit or a need for comfort, follow your plan. You'll find many methods to avoid sugar cravings – find some that work for you. (See page 24).

4. Force the mind to think about something else, just as one of my patients did to resist her cravings for heroin. She focused on 'the opposite' in the situation. If she was sitting, she got up. If she was inside, she went outside for a walk. Call a friend – after a nice 10-minute chat, the sugar craving is gone. Find an activity that makes you happy – jump on a trampoline with the kids, or go bowling. Have some smart snacks ready in the fridge – they may look like desserts but they count as greens, and they calm the sugar craving when you know you are reaching breaking point.

5. Teach yourself to listen to the body's needs, and don't condemn yourself. Ask yourself the following question: 'Why am I standing here with a packet of cookies (or chocolate, or ice cream) again? What genuine need do I have that I hope the cookies will solve? Do I need to calm my stress levels? Do I need comforting, more happiness, entertainment or a reward?' Write down your thoughts and feelings about the situation. Think about what could replace the cookies. If you're stressed, yoga with relaxing music or a quiet 'home spa' can actually remove the need for sweet biscuits. Repeat the exercise whenever needed. Gradually you will get an insight into what you really need, and therefore introduce habits that both body and soul can enjoy. Sugar cravings are an impulse, and by thinking through each situation, the craving is already partially defeated.

6. Introduce a treat day! At our house, Saturday is the day to indulge ourselves with some sweets (candy), ice cream, white bread, white rice sushi, pasta, and so on. Then the mind stops yearning for forbidden fruit – you can look forward to when it can be enjoyed on the next treat day. With increased knowledge about nutrients, you may even find that you make smarter food choices – even on a treat day.

WITH TIME, YOUR INNER MOTIVATION GETS YOU THROUGH

In order for you to succeed, there are some important questions you should answer honestly and sincerely. Do you like your own appearance? How do you see your body shape or your waist? What are the advantages of having a slimmer waist? Do you have any concerns in terms of your weight? Which strengths do you have that you can use to your advantage now that you are making the choice to prepare and eat food that can reduce your waist size? On a scale from 1 to 10, how interested are you in really trying? Can you see any obstacles, and do you have solutions for them? On a scale from 1 to 10, how sure are you that you will try to follow the step-by-step program in this book? On which date will you start? How will you achieve it? Do you need support? How can you seek motivation along the way? Do you have anyone who can do it with you?

Sit down and write a list of why *you* want this so badly. Write down what your goal is. Imagine reaching that target. Say to yourself: 'I look forward to having a 75 cm (29½ inch) waist' or 'I look forward to buying a dress that shows off my waist' or 'I look forward to being able to fit into my own wedding dress again.' Only then will you be able to find the motivation to succeed. On the way, you'll get a helping hand from your inner self. Take a look at your answers when you feel the need. Reward yourself each and every one of the 12 weeks. You are doing this for *yourself* and no one else, because you deserve it!

Don't be too hard on yourself. Appreciate yourself.
You are a unique human being, with your own strengths and vulnerabilities.
You succeed best by being your own best friend.

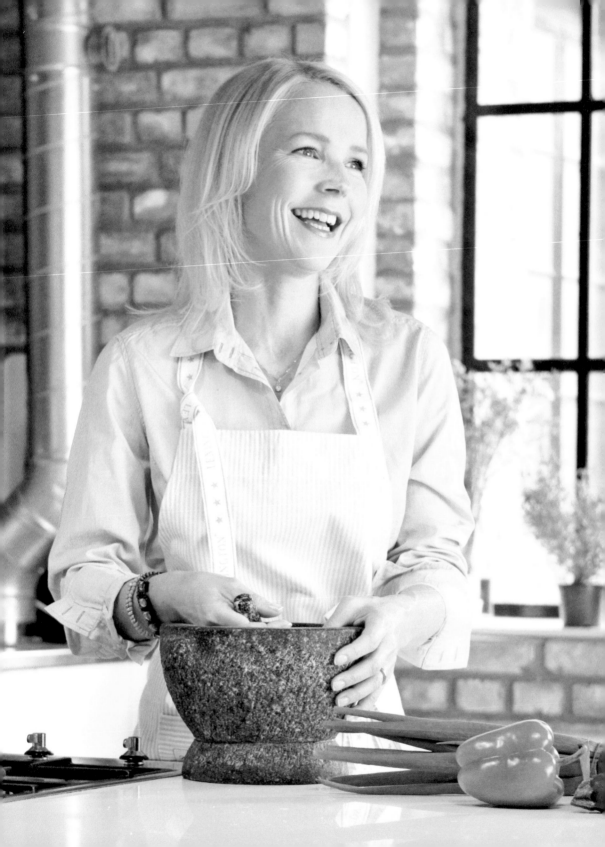

HOW TO USE THIS BOOK

This book describes some simple steps that are implemented week by week over a period of 12 weeks. This is not a diet but a method that creates lasting change in your eating habits for the long term, so that you can maintain good health and a stable ideal weight for the rest of your life. Methods that entail a radical shift in diet overnight will only work for the super-motivated, while a gradual reorganisation is easier to achieve, because you will quickly see the effects of even the simplest little step. It creates curiosity, optimism and motivation, which will make your lifestyle change a lasting success.

Buy yourself a little notebook and write down which goal you are setting yourself. Note your weight and waist size week by week. Decide to allow yourself a bonus for every stepping stone that you reach on the way to achieving your goal. If you want to reduce your weight by 10 kg (22 lb), do something nice for yourself for every second kilo that you lose. Don't worry if the weight is slow to come off. Muscles weigh more than fat, so a remodelling of your body will not necessarily show immediate results on the scales. The important thing is that the dangerous belly fat disappears!

The first four weeks of this 12-week program contain the most important and most effective steps. During these weeks you will stop eating refined white calories, and move over to a daily diet with essential nutrients for mind and body. In the weeks that follow you will learn how the health benefits, weight loss and waist size can be further improved. The last four weeks suggest more tweaks to the method. You'll get tips on the pleasure and enjoyment of food that make it easy to continue on the same path, even after you have reached the waist size that you want.

There are recipes that belong to each chapter and to each week of the book. However, all the recipes can be used at all times, no matter which week you are in. Delicious food is not just recommended for the 12 weeks that are covered in the book. These are recipes for your new life.

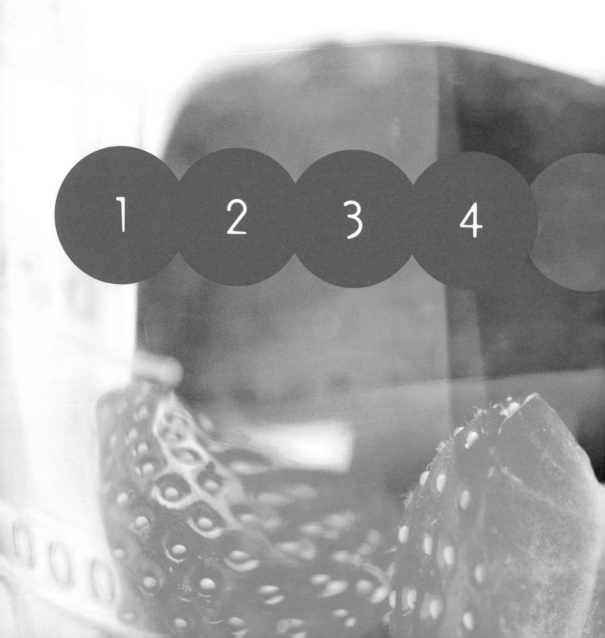

WEEKS 1–4

The first four weeks of this program will give you an insight into the most effective dietary advice to increase the burning of belly fat. Replace the refined white calories that encourage fat storage with delicious alternatives from nature. Take advantage of the latest medical research into foods that reduce your waistline, increase the sensation of fullness and prevent disease.

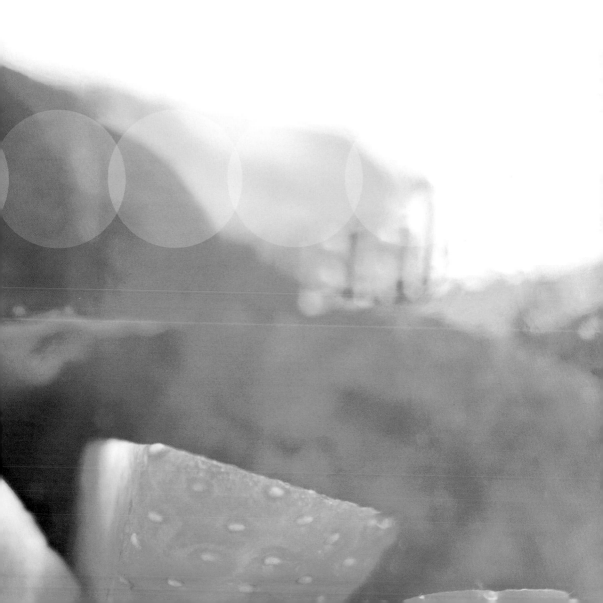

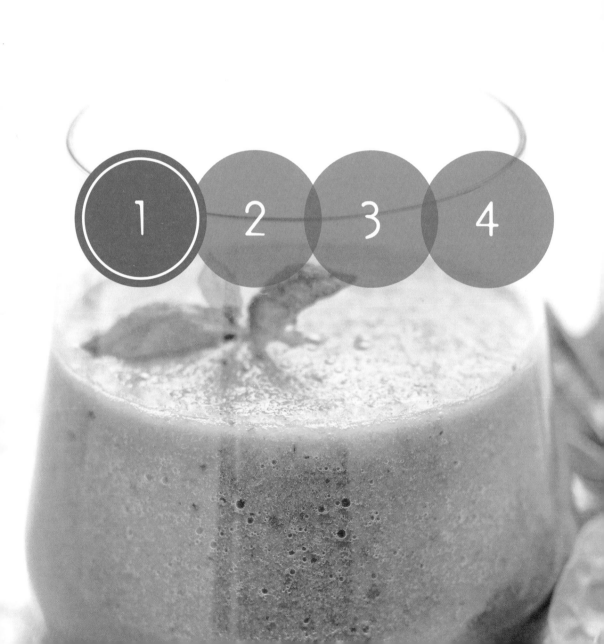

GOAL FOR WEEK 1

This week's exercise is to replace all white sugar, and all products with 'added sugar' shown on the list of ingredients, with the sweet taste of nature. You will be pleasantly surprised by the wonderful flavours that reveal themselves.

Use natural sweeteners

You will achieve the greatest, most decisive effect on waist size by excluding white sugar from your diet. This is because white sugar is easily stored as fat around the stomach. By totally cutting out your consumption of white sugar, both your sweet cravings and your waist size will quickly retreat. Let me explain why. Carbohydrates are absorbed in the intestine and are transformed into glucose, which the brain, muscles and liver can burn as energy. When we eat refined white sugar, this absorption and burning happens very quickly. Blood sugar increases dramatically. Carbohydrates from berries, other fruit and whole wheat are packed inside fibre, proteins and other beneficial nutrients, and this packaging ensures that it takes significantly longer for the body to absorb the sugar and convert it to glucose.

So white sugar is passed at lightning speed from the intestine to the body's cells. Natural carbohydrates, on the other hand, must be divided and separated before they gradually pass into the blood, and this process takes time. It's a much smarter way to fuel the body with energy.

GLUCOSE, INSULIN AND FAT RESERVES

It is important for the body's many organs to get a steady supply of glucose that can be burned as energy. Too much or too little glucose will disrupt the functioning of the vital organs. The body is therefore equipped with sensitive glucose controls. White sugar pushes glucose levels up in sky-high spikes, sounding the body's blood sugar alarm.

When the blood sugar alarm rings, huge supplies of insulin are released to bring the body back into balance. Insulin is the 'key' that unlocks the doors to the body's cells so that glucose can enter – but it is also a fat-storing hormone. When you eat white sugar, you turn off the fat burning and thus store fat. Refraining from eating sugar will also result in less body fat. White sugar is cheap and is found in many food products, not least in drinks.

Studies show that the regular consumption of soft drinks shuts off fat burning and causes both children and adults to be overweight (Collinson 2010, Brown 2008).

When my own blood sugar alarm rings, I become restless, unfocused and irritable. Faced with that situation when I was young, I would dive into my snack drawer. These days I get my fix from nuts and dark chocolate. That's because, throughout my life, I have found that the snack drawer only gives a moment of satisfaction, while nuts give hours of nourishment. Sugar still has the same effect on me – I have just taught myself to be aware of it. Now I choose cakes or biscuits in situations where I feel satisfied and in a good mood – and in limited quantities. *One* piece of cake, not two …

Sugar cravings

Sugar cravings are triggered by blood sugar spikes, persistent alarms and powerful sugar crashes. Context is also important – they can be set off by anxiety, stress or a need for comfort. We all have different sensitivities. Maybe you suffer more sugar cravings than others? Regardless of your situation, there are great benefits to be gained in mood, energy and health by cutting out sugar.

High blood sugar peaks stun the binding sites, also called receptors, in the cells that register sweetness. Therefore your body will constantly seek more sweetness in order to satisfy itself. This leaves you with a body that grows hungrier and hungrier for sugar!

And that's not all. White sugar is stripped of virtually all vitamins, minerals and plant nutrients – nutrients that are used up when sugar burns as energy. In reality you are not only eating 'empty calories', but are also being drained of nutrients. Even if you burn enough *calories* on a treadmill so that your 'calorie account' gets back to zero, the account goes negative when it comes to *nutrients*.

Even if you totally cut out white sugar from your daily life, you can still indulge in a piece of chocolate or a slice of cake once in a while. Your sensitivity for sweet things will be at the front of your mind and you will feel content with much less sweetness than before. A cup of fruit or herbal tea suddenly becomes sweet enough, even without sugar.

SLOW CARBOHYDRATES FOR A SLIMMER WAIST

Starting in week 1 you will treat yourself with sweetness from natural sources, with slow carbohydrates. The slow carbohydrates are absorbed slowly in the intestines and provide a steadily rising, long-lasting and stable level of blood sugar. Such foods do not overload your body with blood sugar alarms. We call them foods with low *glycaemic index* (GI). Apples, pears, plums, nectarines and berries have low glycaemic indexes. All types of vegetables are also included – when you roast them, you'll discover that they have a wonderful sweetness.

Did you know that large swings in blood sugar increase the secretion of the stress hormone cortisol, which in turn encourages fat to be stored around the belly?

When you choose slow carbohydrates from fruits and berries, you achieve stable blood sugar, more energy, lower anxiety, less stress, a better sensation of fullness, a smaller waist size and a more consistent ideal weight. These carbohydrates also help to improve sleep at night and strengthen the helpful bacteria in the gut. They are great benefits that come from a relatively simple change.

Not convinced? Imagine that those spikes in glucose transform the blood sugar into a syrup that attaches to proteins, fatty acids and other nutrients that are carried in the bloodstream. Nutrients with a sugar coating change their properties – yes, they more easily stick to the artery walls. Just think how your feet stick to the floor when somebody has spilled a soft drink. The effect is more or less the same. Sugar-coated nutrients can create a big mess in your body. They can trigger inflammation, encourage water retention, drain you of energy and promote wrinkled skin. Indeed, after the sweet taste comes the bitter sting …

Choose slow, natural carbohydrates – enjoy the taste, and a shrinking waist!

Replace white sugar with honey – a sweetener with smart nutrients

I add half a teaspoon of honey to a cup of plain yoghurt or in warm milk – or add a little honey to a homemade breakfast cereal. It's a perfect complement to the flavours and, rather wonderfully, it's the perfect complement to your health. Honey was a well-known medicine for our ancestors, and is now being rediscovered as a way to soothe throats and heal wounds. Today we also know that sweet tastes stimulate neurotransmitters in the brain's reward centre – dopamine, serotonin and endorphins. As opposed to white sugar, honey contains a number of smart nutrients. The interaction between the enzymes, amino acids, minerals, vitamins, flavours and many plant nutrients of this extraordinary sweetener provide health-boosting benefits.

Even if the GI in honey varies between different types (32–85), after consumption of a single tablespoon (25 g or 1 oz) of most types of honey, GI is low. Actually, several sugars in honey have an extremely low GI and contribute to stable blood sugar and to improved burning of fat (van Can 2009).

Moderate daily use of honey has proven to be favourable to the levels of blood sugar and cholesterol, the immune system and body weight (Yaghoobi 2008). Moreover, honey can reduce the level of inflammatory substances in your body. One study shows that inflammatory substances were reduced by more than 50% after just two weeks (Bogdanov 2008). So, get your hands on some of this amazing sweetener and make sure you take a teaspoonful daily.

Good advice

✳ Remove refined sugars from your cupboards and drawers and buy many different types of honey. Choose flavours that you like, the least refined possible, in order to get the most nutrients possible. Personally I like flower honey, but not heather honey. Acacia honey has an even milder taste than flower honey. Daily intake should depend on your energy use (1 teaspoon to 1 tablespoon per day). Keep honey in a cool, dark place and eat it when it is fresh – after six months of storage, the level of antioxidants can be reduced by up to 30%.

✳ From now on, use a little honey in dishes that you would usually sprinkle with sugar, such as porridge and other breakfast cereal, or in tea.

✳ Cut out sugar in coffee. It's better to soften coffee with a little milk and sprinkle ½ teaspoon of ground cinnamon into the cup.

✳ Note situations where you feel the need for sweetness, and plan a different treat like nuts or dark chocolate, fruit salad or other smart desserts, green tea, coffee or vegetables and dips. See beritnordstrand.no for more tips.

✳ Keep your hands busy when watching TV. A mug of tea or some handicrafts can make you eat less.

✳ Read the contents label on all food products. Breakfast cereals, bread, juice and yoghurt can contain many spoonfuls of sugar. Some kinds of yoghurt can contain more sugar than soft drinks!

✳ *Eat* fruit and berries – don't *drink* them in the form of juice with food. The consumption of fruit juice should be limited to 100–150 ml (3½–5 fl oz) and preferably enjoyed as a snack along with other fruit.

✳ Don't use artificial sweeteners. Studies show that they can increase your sweet cravings and discourage fat burning so that you store more fat around the waist (cf. Nettleton, Diabetes Care 2009).

✳ Be aware that white or refined sugar is not always shown as an ingredient in food products. It can be presented under false names such as glucose, glucose syrup, fructose, syrup or fructose syrup. If you see that a food product contains one of these ingredients, simply choose something else.

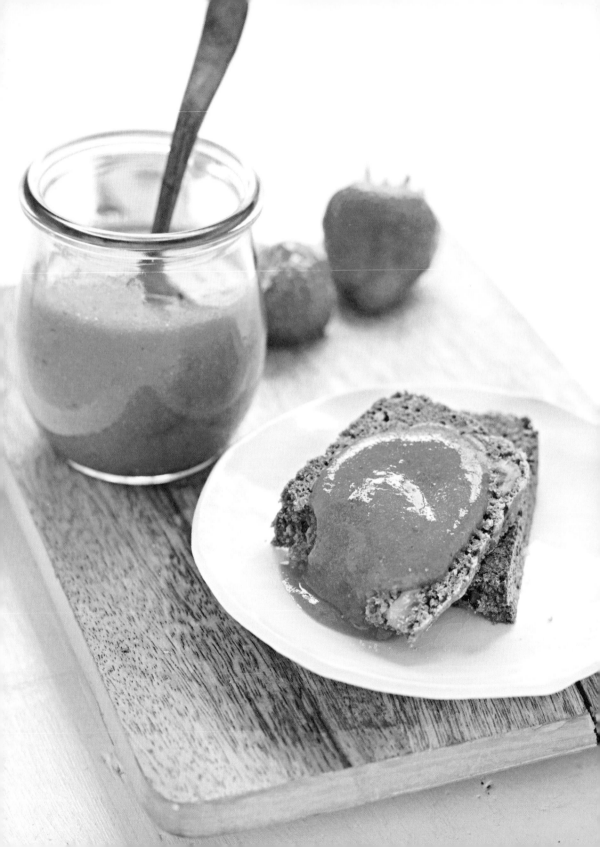

Jam from the blender

This jam is free from sugar and additives, yet packed with flavour and nutrients. The pectin from the apple stiffens the jam, even without additives.

MAKES 200–300 ML (7–10½ FL OZ)

500 g (1 lb 2 oz) berries (a mix of different colourful berries, such as
  strawberries, raspberries, redcurrants or blueberries)
½ unpeeled apple, coarsely chopped

Blend the berries and apple together at full speed to a smooth purée.
Stir the jam just before serving. It will keep in an airtight container in the fridge for up to 1 week.

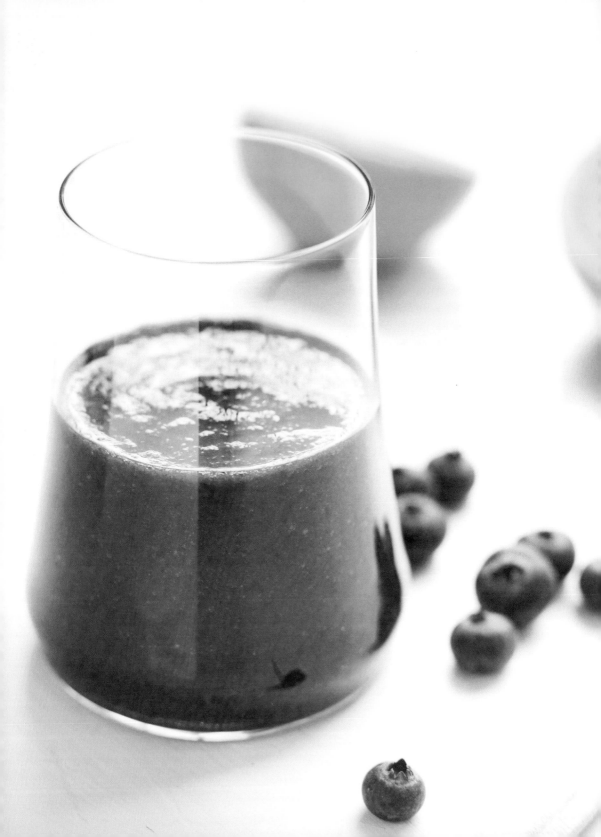

Blueberry and kiwi smoothie

This intensely flavoured smoothie has important nutrients from berries and other fruit.

SERVES 4

2 kiwi fruit
200 g (7 oz) frozen blueberries
1 banana
1 orange, diced
100 ml (3½ fl oz) apple juice (not from concentrate), if you'd like a sweeter smoothie

Put the kiwi fruit, blueberries, banana, orange and apple juice (if using) in a blender, and process to a smooth, even consistency.

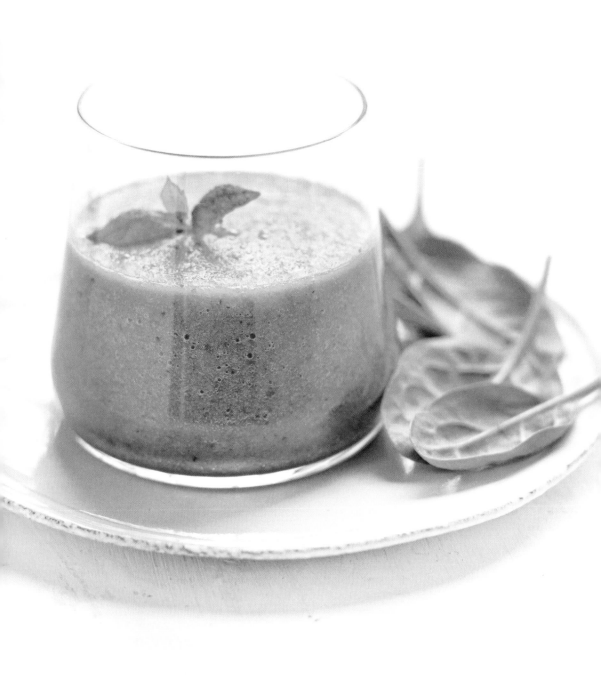

Supergreen smoothie

Full of antioxidants, this delicious smoothie features the wonderful flavours of fruit and green vegetables.

SERVES 4

1 small handful fresh lemon balm leaves
1 celery stalk
½ cucumber
1 apple
1 orange or 2–3 mandarins, or 75 ml (2½ fl oz) orange juice
100 g (3½ oz) baby English spinach
200 ml (7 fl oz) cold water
1 tablespoon grated ginger
2 teaspoons maple syrup

Roughly chop the lemon balm, and cut the celery, cucumber and apple into cubes.
Peel the orange and separate into segments.
Run the spinach, lemon balm, celery, cucumber and water in a blender at full speed for 1–2 minutes until you get a smooth, even consistency. Add the apple, orange, ginger and maple syrup, and blend again until smooth.

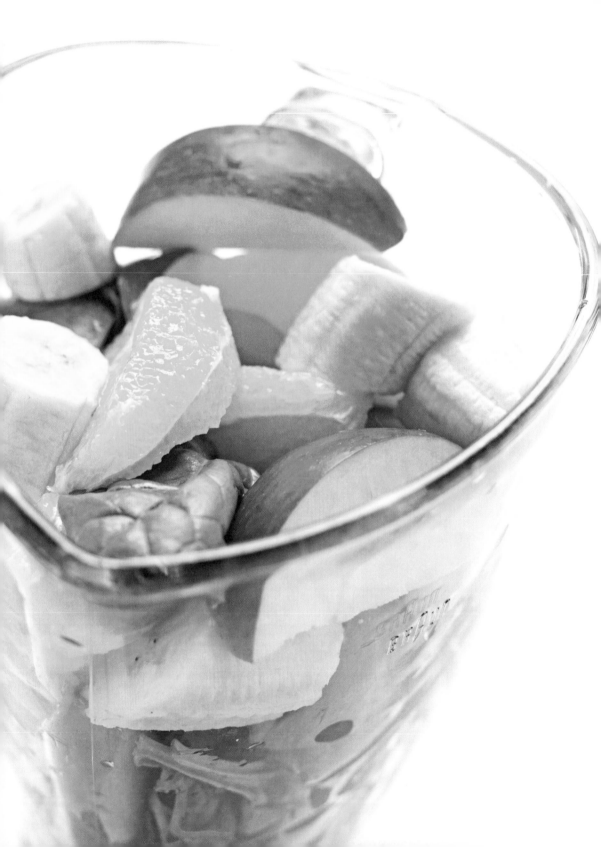

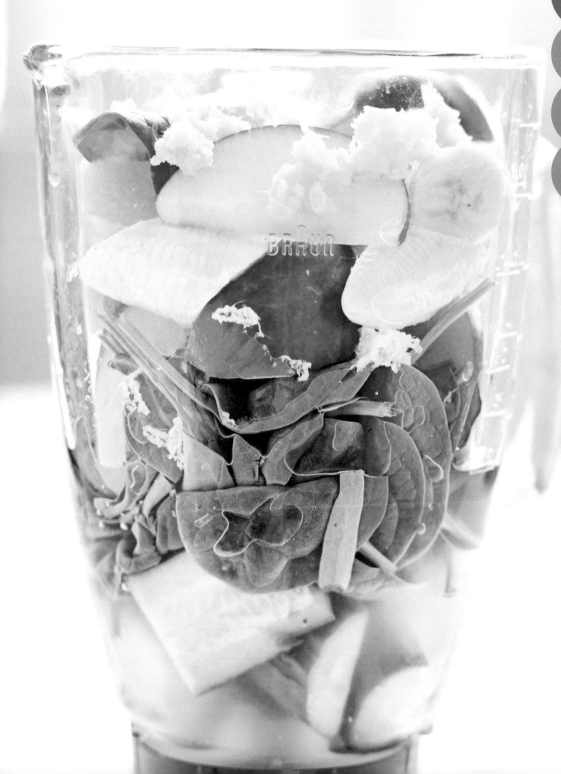

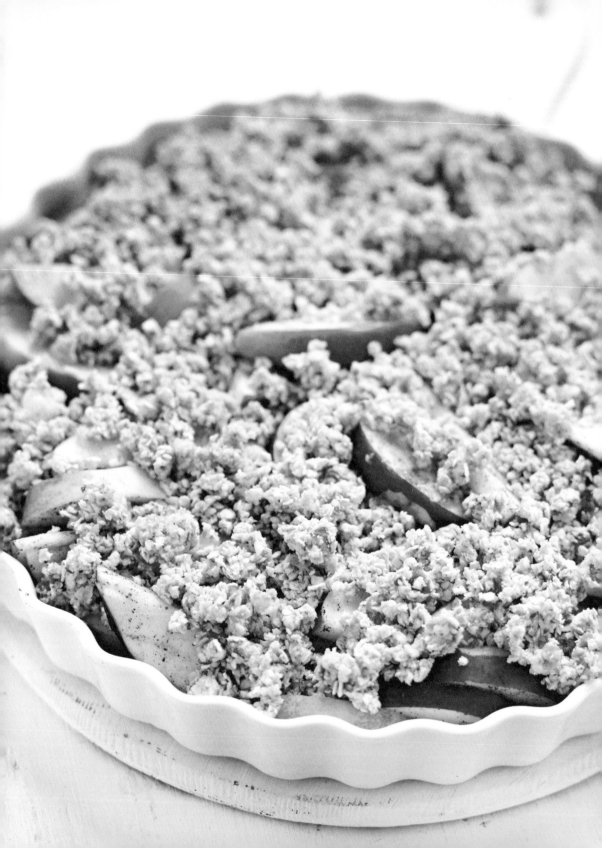

Crumble cake

Crumble cake is quick to make, and the results are almost always great, no matter how you play with the recipe. Gluten and dairy free, it tastes lovely and fresh.

SERVES 8

APPLE FILLING
3 apples, quite sour
2 teaspoons ground cinnamon
seeds from ½ vanilla bean
pinch of ground nutmeg
1 teaspoon honey

TOPPING
50 g (1¾ oz/½ cup) pecans, finely chopped
100 g (3½ oz) gluten-free, quick rolled (porridge) oats
1 tablespoon almond meal or other ground nuts (optional)
1 tablespoon organic coconut oil
1 teaspoon honey or maple syrup

To prepare the apple filling, cut the apple into thin slices, keeping the skin on.
In a mixing bowl, combine all the ingredients. Transfer the filling to a greased ovenproof dish.
Preheat the oven to 175°C (350°F).
Mix all the topping ingredients with your fingers. (You can use a blender or a stick blender if you prefer.) Work the topping together into small crumbs and sprinkle them over the apple filling.
Put the crumble in the oven for 20–30 minutes. The cooking time varies from oven to oven and according to the cake's thickness, but when the filling bubbles and the topping begins to turn golden brown, it's ready. Enjoy!

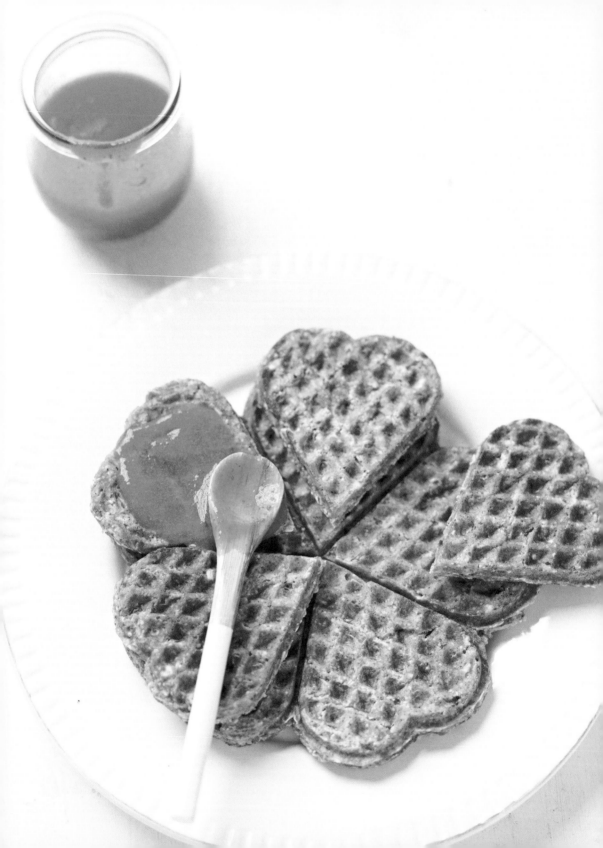

Wholemeal waffles with apple and cinnamon

These home-made waffles give you lots of health-boosting fibre, vitamins, minerals, antioxidants and healthy dairy fats. Put them in an airtight container in the fridge and take some waffle love to school or work with you. You'll need an electric waffle maker for this recipe.

MAKES 2 LARGE WAFFLES

1 apple
200 g (7 oz) quick rolled (porridge) oats
200 g (7 oz) wholemeal (whole-wheat) rye flour
1 teaspoon ground cinnamon
1 egg
1 tablespoon sour cream
2 tablespoons melted butter
100 ml (3½ fl oz) milk
100 ml (3½ fl oz) apple juice

Grate the apple, leaving the skin on. Combine the oats, rye flour and cinnamon in a mixing bowl. In a separate bowl, combine the egg, sour cream, melted butter, milk, apple juice and grated apple, and then stir in the dry ingredients until you have a smooth, even waffle batter.
Spoon half the batter into the waffle machine and cook until browned. Repeat with the remaining batter, keeping the cooked waffle warm.

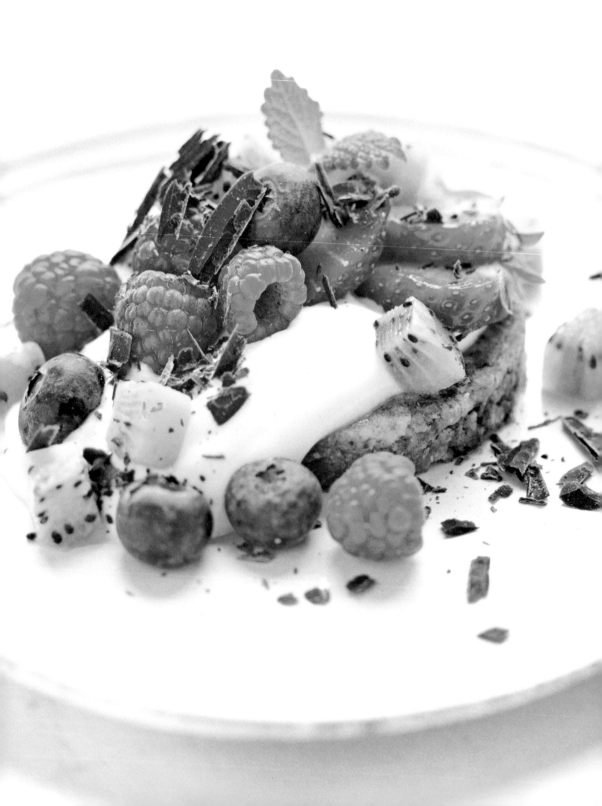

Nut cake

This is a wonderful cake that does not require baking. It contains neither gluten nor dairy products.

SERVES 6

500 g (1 lb 2 oz) nuts and seeds, such as almonds, walnuts, hazelnuts or pepitas (pumpkin seeds)
5 fresh dates or prunes, stones removed
100 g (3½ oz) raisins
2 teaspoons ground cinnamon
¼ teaspoon ground nutmeg
1 teaspoon vanilla powder (optional)
pinch of sea salt
1 tablespoon maple syrup or honey (flower honey is best)

Process half of the nuts and seeds in a blender, until quite finely ground. Repeat with the rest of the nuts and seeds. Transfer all the blended nuts and seeds to a mixing bowl.
Put the dates and raisins in the blender and run it at full speed until they are finely chopped. Mix the cinnamon, nutmeg, vanilla powder and sea salt into the blended nuts, and stir in the chopped dates and raisins.
Drizzle over the maple syrup or honey. Bring the dough together with your fingers.
Press out the dough in a cake shape that measures approximately 22 cm (8½ inches) in diameter, or press it out into six small portions.

TOPPING SUGGESTIONS
- plain yoghurt, fresh fruit, dark chocolate flakes and lemon balm, mint or chervil
- sour cream, softened cranberries and lemon balm, mint or chervil
- sour cream and oven-baked apple slices with ground cinnamon
- fresh blueberries and 2 pears simmered until tender in 200 ml (7 fl oz) apple juice, then diced
- 100 g (3½ oz) melted dark chocolate and 1 tablespoon organic coconut butter, combined to make a chocolate sauce

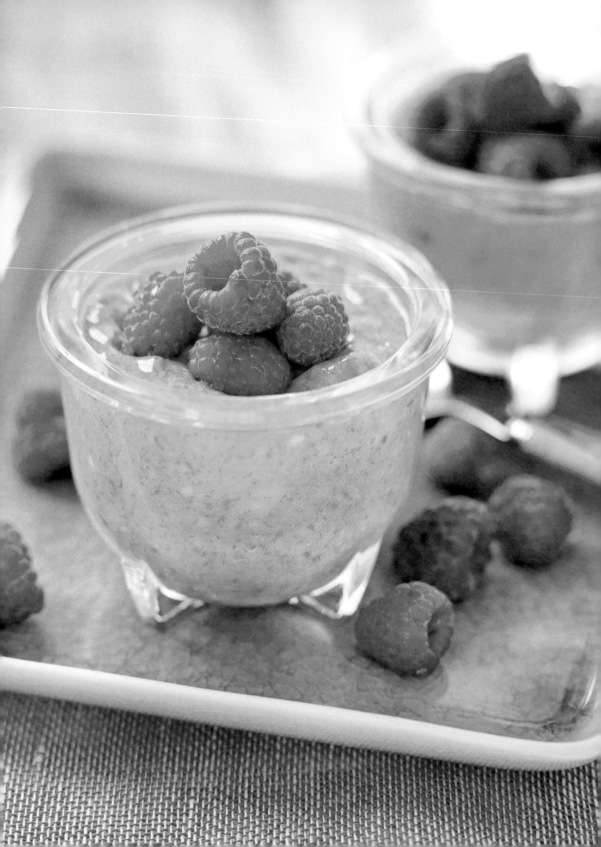

Quick raspberry sorbet from the blender

SERVES 2

½ well-ripened avocado, skin and stone removed
½ frozen banana
200 g (7 oz) frozen raspberries
1 egg
1 tablespoon maple syrup
fresh raspberries, to garnish

Combine the avocado, banana, frozen raspberries, egg and maple syrup in a bowl, and blend with a stick blender until everything is well combined. You can also use a standmixer, but then you will have to stop the mixer a few times and stir by hand to make sure everything is evenly blended. To serve, simply fill two bowls with the raspberry sorbet, decorate with a few fresh raspberries, and enjoy the moment.

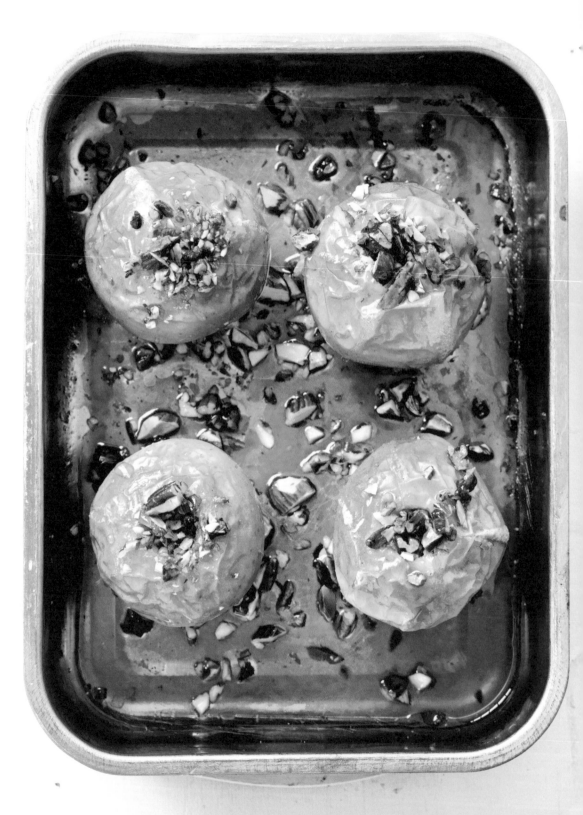

Oven-baked apples

In the same way that roasting root vegetables brings out their naturally sweet flavour, sour apples turn sweet when they are baked in the oven.

SERVES 4

4 apples
1 handful almonds (or any other nuts you have), coarsely chopped
1 handful raisins, coarsely chopped
4 tablespoons maple syrup
plain yoghurt, to serve (optional)

Preheat the oven to 175°C (350°F).
Wash the apples and remove the cores. Cut off a slice from the bottom so that they sit flat in an ovenproof dish.
Fill the holes left by the cores with nuts and raisins, and pour over the maple syrup. Bake in the oven for 40 minutes, or until the apples are tender and a beautiful colour. Serve as they are or with a dash of yoghurt.

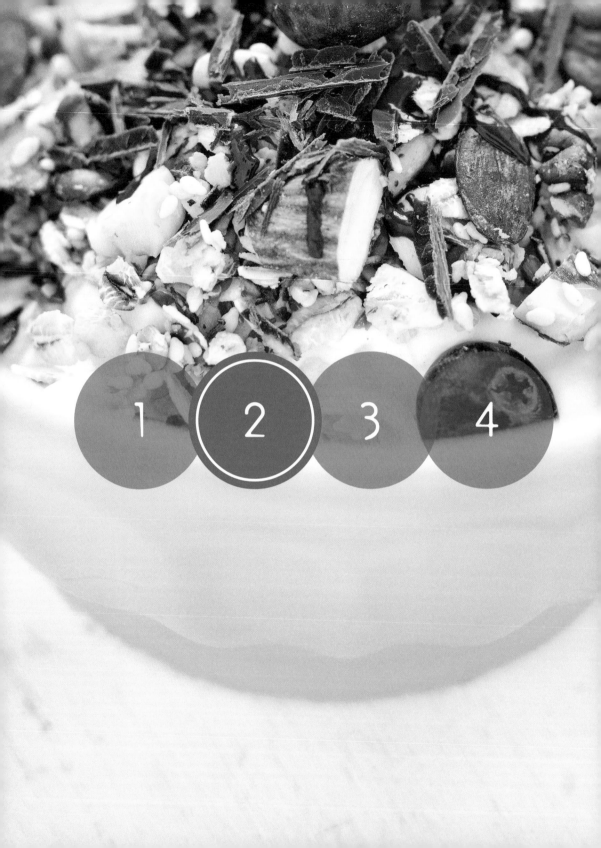

GOAL FOR WEEK 2

The exercise this week is to replace flour-based baked goods with whole grain and seeded breads. The bran and wheat germ from nutritious whole grains gives your baking a wonderful flavour, while increasing both calorie burning and weight loss.

EAT WHOLE GRAINS AND SEEDS

Now that you have made it through the first week, I hope that it feels good to have replaced refined sugars with natural sweetness. This week we are going to focus on the baked goods that we eat. There are many advantages to replacing white bread (baked with refined ingredients, especially white flour) with bread that is baked with whole grains. The following tips offer great-tasting alternatives that will make your baked treats much healthier.

In general we eat far too much refined and fine-grained flour, in which heavy processing has removed or destroyed beneficial nutrients such as fibre, vitamins, minerals, amino acids, fatty acids and plant nutrients that you normally find in whole grains. The flour comes from a grain variety that was developed more to suit the needs of industrial bakers than our need for wholesome nutrients. We are left with baked goods that provide us with more starch, stronger gluten and less nutrition. Starch has more or less the same effect on your body as refined sugar.

We all know how easy it can be to consume refined and fine-grained flours. The aroma of fresh pastries hits me when I'm paying for a drink at the coffee shop in the hospital, and it is followed by the smell of freshly baked focaccia when I'm choosing a salad for lunch.

Chocolate muffins from the coffee stall were the last things one of my patients wanted to give up … so she came up with a little experiment. She sucked on a piece of dark chocolate as she walked into the coffee shop. Then she bought a coffee without sugar, but with steamed milk and a little cinnamon. On the way to that day's consultation she marched past the muffins in style, and collected her reward later with more energy and fewer kilos. A few days later she wanted more smart food tricks. She gradually phased out diet soft drinks in favour of carbonated mineral water and sugar-free pastilles and a handful of nuts. A short while later, she reflected on the experience: 'I think I was addicted to muffins as if they were heroin!' Sugar is a strong addiction with powerful cravings. But read on – you will discover that a daily life free from cakes and soft drinks is easier to achieve than you think, and your days will be much more pleasurable.

Carbohydrates in the form of natural sugars and starches can affect both body weight and mood, but are not harmful in themselves. At a time when trendy diets almost create a hysteria with their condemnation of carbohydrates, it is easy to forget that carbs also have important functions for the body. The brain, liver and muscles all prefer nourishment of this type, and the brain alone burns around 120–130 g (4¼–4½ oz) of carbohydrates every single day.

A CARBOHYDRATE IS NOT JUST A CARBOHYDRATE

It is not just white sugar that contributes to sky-high spikes in blood sugar and reduced fat burning. Some natural sugars and starches in natural ingredients can also be absorbed quickly in the intestine and create big spikes in blood sugar. Then unnatural amounts of blood sugar attach themselves to the blood vessel walls and, from there, are on their way through the bloodstream.

Sugar clings to proteins in the brain, eyes, bloodstream and muscles, and can affect their functioning. Being soaked in sugar like this has been associated with dementia, high blood pressure, cardiovascular disease, diabetes, poor eyesight and premature ageing. These sticky proteins are called, a little vividly, AGE (Advanced Glycosylated End-products). Preventing the production of AGE is therefore both health-boosting and revitalising.

Slow carbohydrates, on the other hand, have to be processed in the intestine before they can be absorbed. Over time, they provide a slowly rising and stable blood sugar level. With slow carbohydrates the blood sugar never becomes so high that it is harmful. You will find these carbohydrates in vegetables, whole grains, brown rice, berries and other fruit. They offer great nutrients, and they never settle around the waist. So it's crazy to avoid all forms of carbohydrates – avoid those that are absorbed quickly in the intestine, and stick to the slow, beneficial ones.

You can cut down significantly on the amount of fast carbohydrates if you avoid foods that are made of wheat. White bread, refined crackers, most breakfast cereals, pastries and biscuits, pasta and white rice are some of the foods you ought to steer clear of. You should also avoid foods that are labelled 'added sugar', but you have already done that, haven't you?

SEVEN GREAT SOURCES OF SLOW CARBOHYDRATES FROM WHOLE GRAINS

(ASSUMING THEY ARE UNSWEETENED)

1 rye bread
2 wholegrain bread
3 wholegrain crackers
4 rolled (porridge) oats
5 steel-cut oats
6 barley oats
7 wholegrain muesli

What is the link between fast carbohydrates and the amount of belly fat? The key word is insulin. This is a hormone that releases glucose into the cells. When you eat fast carbohydrates, you experience a big spike in blood sugar. As I'm sure you know from last week, that means that the body sends out an alarm that the blood sugar is too high and therefore produces insulin to release the sugar into the cells so that they can use them as fuel. High blood sugar leads to the production of batches of insulin in order to restore the balance. But the mechanism overshoots the target, blood sugar drops a little too quickly and that triggers a new type of alarm. Now blood sugar has become too low. Hunger and sugar cravings strike as the body strives to raise the blood sugar in order to guarantee delivery to cells in their billions.

The liver also contributes to keeping the blood sugar low by storing a little sugar and converting glucose into fat. The insulin hormone opens the fat cells so that fat can be stored. The fat cells in the belly, in particular, are sensitive to insulin and open up easily. Refined carbohydrates therefore settle around the waist. So every time you produce insulin, you flip the belly's fat-storing switch.

Think about insulin as a double-edged sword. It's both a vital friend and a potential foe. The goal is a stable and steady level – always enough, but never too much. As with so much else in the body, it's about balance – just enough is perfect, but too much or too little simply will not work.

Studies have shown that factors such as too much sitting, being overweight, smoking, the consumption of hydrogenated fats, a lack of sleep and stress can increase insulin production. This is because the cells' sensitivity to insulin is reduced, so more insulin has to be produced in order for the cells to allow glucose in. These factors, along with fast carbohydrates, contribute to the steady increase of fat storage around the waist. Moving a little more, quitting smoking, avoiding hydrogenated fat, sleeping enough and stressing a little less will increase insulin sensitivity while the amount of belly fat goes into decline. By taking these steps and cutting down on fast carbohydrates, you will achieve fabulous results.

The hormone that says no!

Slow carbohydrates from fibre-rich vegetables, nuts, seeds and whole grains have a positive effect on fat burning by increasing the production of a hormone that you have probably never heard about: adiponectin. Think about it as a hormone that refuses to let fat settle around the waist. Studies show that the hormone actually increases the rate of fat burning (Qi 2006).

But it is, nevertheless, important that you steer clear of fast carbohydrates. Big spikes in insulin from fast carbohydrates actually weaken your body's production of adiponectin (Kelesidis 2006).

Lower levels of the fat-burning hormone adiponectin have been measured in studies of the overweight, especially in overweight people with a large waist measurement. Low adiponectin is also associated with the increased occurrence of type-2 diabetes, high blood pressure, cardiovascular disease, metabolic syndrome and cancer.

Limit the bread you eat

Studies show that eating equal proportions of protein, fat and slow carbohydrates gives you a slimmer waist, builds muscle mass and delivers a more resilient body (Wycherley 2010). In order to achieve this balance on your plate, you can cut slices of bread a little thinner and be a bit more generous with salad leaves, cucumber slices, tomatoes and toppings of deli meat, fish, egg and cheese.

FORMULA FOR A BALANCED OPEN SANDWICH

IT'S TIME FOR THE TOPPINGS AND GREENS TO DOMINATE YOUR PLATE!

1. One slice of wholemeal (whole wheat) bread (for example, rye bread or similar)
2. A thin spread of butter, mayonnaise, hummus, guacamole, salsa or similar
3. A handful of green salad leaves
4. Some nice pieces of fish (oily fish, such as herring or salmon), meat (such as left-over chicken) or egg
5. Garnish with more vegetables, such as sliced capsicum (pepper), diced avocado or cucumber slices

Good advice when you bake bread in the oven or bread machine

✳ Choose whole grains, preferably organic or stoneground flour. Don't use refined flour.

✳ Mix chopped nuts and seeds into the dough.

✳ Replace some of the wheat flour with flour made from seeds, pulses or nuts (for example, quinoa flour, buckwheat flour, chickpea flour or almond meal). You can find these flours in health food shops.

✳ Add bran and wheat germ to your baking.

✳ Use less yeast and instead let the dough rise for longer (preferably overnight).

✳ Bake the bread at a lower temperature than you're used to, so that you get succulent and nutritious loaves. Try baking at 175°C (350°F) for 1–1½ hours. Cover the bread with foil so it doesn't become too hard.

Take note of when you most often fall into the fast carbs bread trap. Is it at the cafeteria while you're working? When you buy a take-away coffee at the café or when you're out for lunch? Have a box of nuts and a bit of dark chocolate on standby, so it will be easier to resist the temptations. Ask for whole-grain alternatives at the café or restaurant (I politely ask the waiter to remove the bread from the table), or choose salads and soups with good sources of protein such as chicken, fish or egg. In this way you'll get full without eating bread on top. Come up with a good strategy to take control of those situations when you know you'll be tempted by white bread and pastries. Saying 'no thanks' to white bread is a big step in the right direction. I'm cheering you on!

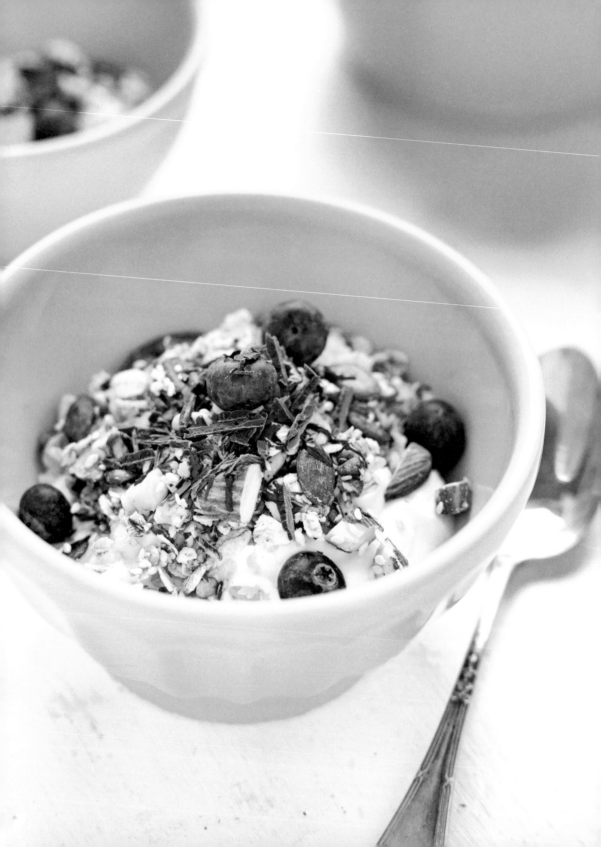

Berit's breakfast cereal

Making your own breakfast cereal is easy – and it tastes much better than most of the ones you can buy at the supermarket. While store-bought cereals can contain as much sugar as a packet of biscuits, this one is sweetened with a little honey.

MAKES ABOUT 1.5 KG (3 LB 5 OZ)

100 g (3½ oz) hazelnuts
100 g (3½ oz) walnuts
100 g (3½ oz) almonds
100 g (3½ oz) linseeds (flaxseeds)
100 g (3½ oz) sunflower seeds
100 g (3½ oz) pepitas (pumpkin seeds)
100 g (3½ oz) sesame seeds
700 g (1 lb 9 oz) quick rolled (porridge) oats
100 g (3½ oz) honey
2½ tablespoons extra virgin olive oil
100 g (3½ oz) shredded coconut and/or 50 g (1¾ oz) chopped dark chocolate (optional)

Preheat the oven to 140°C (275°F).
Chop all the nuts.
Crush the linseeds in a blender.
Combine all the dry ingredients.
Heat the honey and oil in a small saucepan, and stir the blend into the dry ingredients. Mix well.
Divide the mixture between two baking trays lined with baking paper, and spread out.
Bake in the oven for 30–35 minutes, stirring a few times during baking.
Let the mixture cool down, and stir in the coconut and/or the chopped chocolate (if using). You can also stir in more porridge oats, if you like.
Serve with fresh berries and plain yoghurt.

TIP: Add 2 teaspoons ground cinnamon with the honey if you want a cinnamon-flavoured breakfast cereal. In this case, use even more porridge oats to fill out the mixture.

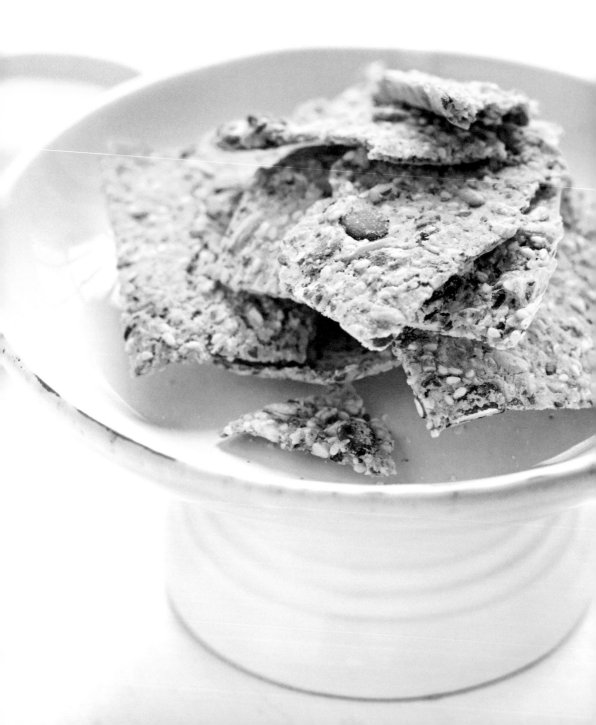

Gluten-free crackers

These gluten-free crackers are packed full of great flavour and nutrients.

100 g (3½ oz) sesame seeds
100 g (3½ oz) linseeds (flaxseeds)
100 g (3½ oz) sunflower seeds
100 g (3½ oz) pepitas (pumpkin seeds)
100 g (3½ oz) pecans or walnuts
800 g (1 lb 12 oz) almond meal
400 g (14 oz) gluten-free, quick rolled (porridge) oats
200 g (7 oz) buckwheat flour
1 teaspoon sea salt
800 ml (28 fl oz) water

Preheat the oven to 175°C (350°F).
Run the seeds quickly through a coffee grinder or blender, so that they are a little crushed. Finely chop the nuts.
Combine all the dry ingredients. Add the water, mix well and let it sit for 20 minutes.
Spread a 2–3 mm (⅟₁₆ –⅛ inch) layer of the mixture evenly over two baking trays covered with baking paper. If the mixture is too thick to spread out, add a little more water.
Bake the crackers in the oven for around 30 minutes. It's better to place both trays in the oven at the same time. Be careful that the crackers don't burn.
Take the trays out when the crackers are still a little soft or half-baked, but hard enough that they can be lifted or moved. Leave the oven door slightly open while you take out the trays and cut up the cracker dough into bite-sized pieces with a pizza cutter.
Turn the temperature down to 100°C (200°F). Return the crackers to the trays and dry in the oven for around 1 hour, with the oven door slightly open.

TIP: When you grind sesame seeds and linseeds, it becomes easier for the body to absorb the nutrients they contain. That's especially important for linseeds. Otherwise, the body can only make use of the fibre in them. The texture of the crackers becomes smoother as well.

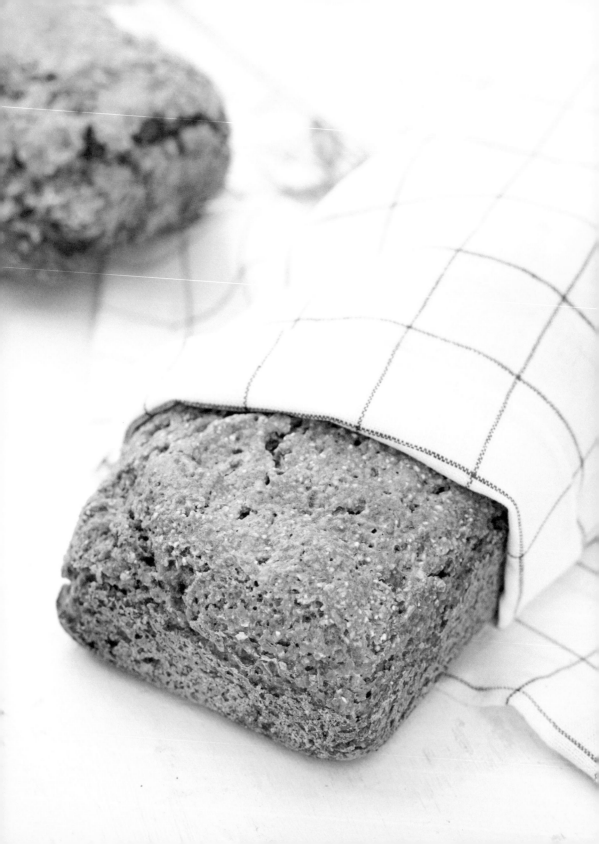

Berit's seed bread

A fantastically nice and simple, no-knead daily bread with loads of nutrients from both whole grains and seeds.

MAKES 2 LOAVES

25 g (1 oz) fresh yeast
1 litre (35 fl oz/4 cups) lukewarm water
1 teaspoon honey
150 g (5½ oz) linseeds (flaxseeds)
480 g (1 lb 1 oz) wholemeal (whole-wheat) spelt flour
480 g (1 lb 1 oz) wholemeal (whole-wheat) rye flour
150 g (5½ oz) pepitas (pumpkin seeds)
150 g (5½ oz) sesame seeds
2 teaspoons salt
1 teaspoon caraway seeds (optional)

Dissolve the yeast in the water, and stir in the honey. Place the linseeds in a blender and blend for 3–4 seconds. Combine all the dry ingredients in a mixing bowl or standmixer. Add the yeast mixture and mix well. The dough should be quite loose.
Put the dough in a warm place away from draughts under a tea towel (dish towel) to rise overnight, around 12 hours.
Divide the dough between two bread tins, either greased or lined with baking paper. Set them aside to rise for 1 hour more.
Preheat the oven to 175°C (350°F), then bake the loaves for 1 hour. Remove from the tins and let them cool down on a cooling rack.

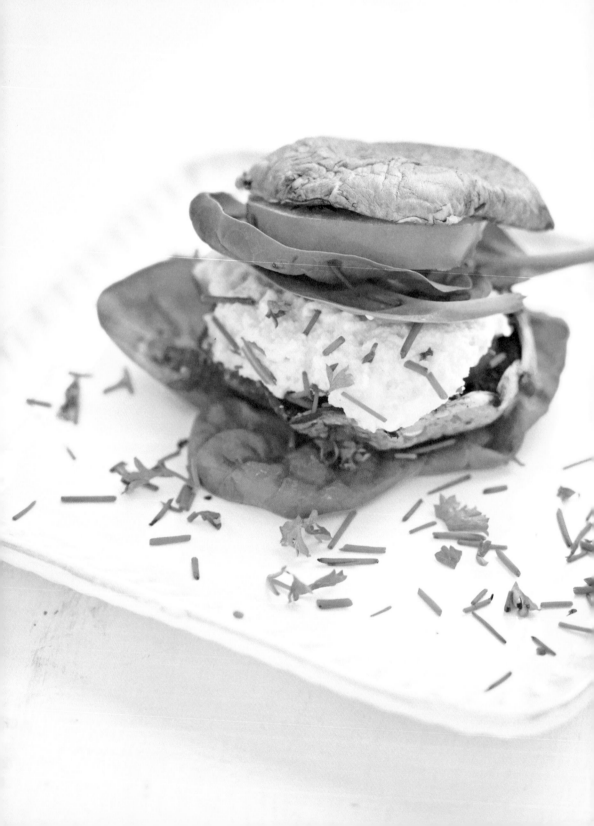

Portobello burger

Portobello mushrooms are classic 'meaty' mushrooms, with a rich, mild flavour. They are both bread and burger in this recipe!

MAKES 2

4 portobello mushrooms
1 tablespoon extra virgin olive oil
1 tablespoon soy sauce
1 handful grated medium–hard cheese (choose your favourite) or vegan cashew mousse
  (see recipe below)
2 tomatoes, sliced
2 tablespoons chopped flat-leaf (Italian) parsley
2 tablespoons chopped chives
lettuce or baby English spinach, to serve … or whatever takes your fancy!

VEGAN CASHEW MOUSSE
250 g (9 oz) cashew nuts, soaked overnight
100 ml (3½ fl oz) water
juice of 1 lemon
1 garlic clove
herbs, such as basil, thyme, oregano or rosemary (optional)

Make the cashew mousse first: put all the ingredients in a blender and process to an even, thick consistency. Place the mousse in the fridge for at least 2 hours. It keeps well for a couple of days. This portion is so large that you can use it in other dishes.
Preheat the oven to 175°C (350°F).
Remove the stalks from the mushrooms. Combine the olive oil and the soy sauce, and brush the mushrooms with the marinade. Repeat the brushing 2–3 times so that the mushrooms absorb the marinade. Put the mushrooms in a small ovenproof dish and bake for 10–15 minutes, until they are soft, dark and smelling wonderful.
When the mushrooms are ready, assemble the burgers by scattering the cheese or cashew mousse over the mushrooms, layering over the tomatoes, scattering over more cheese and then the herbs. Make double-deckers if you like. Put the mushrooms back in the oven, and bake until the cheese melts.
Serve with lettuce or baby English spinach.

GOAL FOR WEEK 3

This week's exercise is to eat more vegetables, berries, herbs and spices. You will learn how many plant nutrients increase fat burning, curb inflammation and slim your waist. Welcome to nature's pantry!

Eat vegetables and increase fat burning

It's great that you're still hanging in there! It's fantastic that you've replaced white sugar with natural sweetness, and that refined white flour has been swapped for whole grains. Your cells are already enjoying the effect of many more nutrients. When nutrients are converted into energy, they produce 'sparks' called free radicals or oxidants. This week you'll get advice on some simple steps and foods that will ensure you don't get burned. Eating plenty of greens is the key.

Nature really knows how to do it – all the world's useful nutrients, which work together and strengthen each other, have been put into a single foodstuff. Vegetables, berries and other fruit provide the power of antioxidants, fibre, fatty acids, protein, slow carbohydrates and a host of vitamins and minerals. Half your plate ought to be filled with this plant power. All you need to do is learn how to prepare vegetables, and how to sneak berries into different dishes, so that they become a delight both for the tastebuds and the body.

An audience member at one of my lectures became motivated by the fact that salad greens have more 'anti-wrinkle effect' than the most expensive face creams. She began to make green smoothies for vanity's sake, but ended up becoming a convert after noticing the significant effect on her mood and energy levels, and on the scales. She was astonished by how a handful of green leaves could have started a process within her that has now given her a whole new life.

Studies show that the metabolism's 'sparks' – *oxidants* – can affect your brain's satiety centre so that it becomes less sensitive to the fullness hormones, so you eat more before you feel full. *Antioxidants* eliminate those sparks and increase sensitivity in the fullness centre, so that you feel full faster. So treat yourself to more antioxidant-rich plant foods, which you'll find among unprocessed herbs, vegetables, berries and other fruit.

Studies have shown that you can reduce your waistline and lose weight by eating *more* – if it's vegetables that you're eating. A six-month study of 80 overweight Brazilians showed that, for every additional 100 g (3½ oz) of vegetables that they ate every day, there was a reduction in weight of 500 g (1 lb 2 oz) (Sartorelli 2008).

Furthermore, a range of studies has shown that an increased intake of fruit and greens promotes weight loss in both adults and children (Ledoux 2011). The weight loss has several causes: vegetables, berries and a variety of other fruits are rich in water and fibre, offer the body a low sugar load, and contain relatively few calories. These can easily replace more calorie-rich food. A study of Spaniards aged 15–80 showed that weight gain during the teenage years was significantly reduced among those who ate a lot of fruit and vegetables (Vioque 2008).

Blueberries are my favourite berries. That's because they taste great and remind me of blueberry hunts, pancakes, Advent and mulled wine. Blueberries are among the most antioxidant-rich fruits and berries that you can find (Wu 2004). They can stamp out 'sparks' from the metabolism, curb the production of inflammatory substances from belly fat cells, improve insulin sensitivity, correct cholesterol levels, speed up fat burning, and reduce the amount of belly fat (Mizuno 2013). But you can also find powerful antioxidants in many other types of colourful berries, so indulge in a little bowl of berries every day. Add coloured berries such as blueberries, cranberries, cloudberries, raspberries and/or strawberries to smoothies and yoghurt, to porridge oats and to salads, too.

Avocado is a fruit that you either love or hate – even if many think of it as a vegetable. I love its creamy texture, its mild taste and, above all, the unsaturated fatty acids, minerals and plant nutrients it offers. My daughter Karoline has to mix it well with salsa so she can eat it. One avocado can give you a total of 10 g (¼ oz) of fibre. Consuming more fibre can lead to a reduction in the amount of inflammatory substances in the blood, more energy, and increased burning of belly fat (Parikh 2012). Avocados are really useful because they don't have a very prominent flavour. They are well suited to adding a creamy texture to chocolate mousse; they are filling and taste great in green salads; and they are good enough alone with some prawn (shrimp) salad and lemon.

HOW YOU CAN GET ENOUGH PLANT ENERGY IN DAILY LIFE

＊ A great rule of thumb is to eat two handfuls of 'rainbow greens' for every handful of protein.

＊ Enjoy a small bowl of colourful berries.

＊ Vary between raw, steamed, boiled and oven-roasted vegetables. Different cooking methods suit the different nutrients. While vitamins are best preserved in raw vegetables, cooking will increase the uptake of simple plant nutrients, such as orange colourants containing antioxidants (carotenoids).

＊ A little extra virgin olive oil, some melted butter or naturally fatty ingredients such as sliced egg, cheese or avocado goes superbly with vegetables. The fat increases the uptake of helpful nutrients.

MORE FIBRE MEANS A SLIMMER WAIST

Fibre is the part of the plant that cannot be broken down in the intestine, but nevertheless is important for the nurturing of bacteria, for digestion and for nutrition. It is the cell walls and plant starch that isn't absorbed by the body. This starch is called resistant starch, and can improve your insulin sensitivity (Johnston 2010), which moderates the need to make insulin in order to allow glucose to enter the cells. Fibre also holds sugar back in the intestine, so that the rate of absorption is slowed, the glucose stays stable and less insulin is required. Less insulin means less fat storage around the waist.

Studies show that this type of starch – which you'll find in beans and lentils, for example – can also increase fat burning and conserve muscle mass during times when you are eating fewer calories and the burning of fat would usually be scaled down. More muscle mass means a faster metabolism and an increased burning of calories, even when you are at rest. When you do strengthening exercises, the effect is increased significantly.

Even in itself, the breaking down of fibre-rich food burns calories without you moving a single muscle. All in all, the consumption of fibre-rich food makes it easier for you to maintain a stable ideal weight (Higgins 2013).

It has been shown that the composition of the ingredients on your dinner plate means far more for hunger, and for fullness after a meal, than the mere calorie count. Hunger is triggered by hunger hormones, and fullness by the fullness hormones. A study showed that protein- and fibre-rich food leads to steadier blood sugar, lower insulin levels and fewer hunger hormones than meals with similar amounts of calories, but less protein and fibre (Karhunen 2010). A modest reduction in fibre intake can lead to significantly more belly fat. More fibre-rich vegetables, therefore, means increased weight loss and a smaller waist (Davis 2009).

HOW YOU CAN GET MORE FIBRE-RICH VEGETABLES IN DAILY LIFE

* Think: two handfuls of vegetables for every handful of animal protein (meat, fish, eggs).

* Aim for 2–3 kinds of different coloured vegetables at every mealtime.

* Eat raw vegetables as a starter or on the side.

* Mix chopped vegetables into cooked barley, lentils and quinoa.

* Add vegetables such as cucumber, celery, spinach leaves, and so on, to smoothies.

* Make vegetable sticks and dip, so you can take them with you in your lunchbox.

* Make vegetable omelettes.

* Make vegetable soups and stir-fries.

IS THERE ANY VALUE IN THE FAMOUS GRAPEFRUIT DIET?

Plant energy doesn't just mean vegetables and berries. Studies show that other fruit can also protect against weight gain (Alinia 2009). In order to avoid insulin surges that inhibit fat burning, select fruit that gives the body a low sugar load (low GI). If you choose apples, pears, plums or nectarines, you can eat almost as much as you like.

You have surely heard about celebrities who start the day with a grapefruit to kickstart fat burning. I remember well when the grapefruit diet was launched at the end of the 1970s. My girlfriends and I threw ourselves at the craze. We didn't know then that the icing (confectioners') sugar that we heaped on top destroyed most of the health-boosting effects. We had misunderstood the grapefruit diet, got bored after a short while and all agreed that bread and cheese was best for breakfast. But a single grapefruit before mealtimes can probably help. A 12-week American study of 91 overweight people showed that half a grapefruit before every main meal produced a weight reduction of 1.6 kg (3 lb 8 oz) compared to about 335 g (11¾ oz) in the control group. Insulin sensitivity was also improved in the grapefruit group. Many researchers now recommend a little fresh grapefruit as a helping hand on the way to a slimmer life.

Your blood sugar spikes will, however, get a little higher if you consume fruit in the form of juice, as the amount of fructose absorbed is much greater than with whole fruit. Eat fruit – don't drink it. This is because an excess of fructose – or fruit sugar – gets converted into fat. It doesn't help if it is all natural sugar – in large doses it will also turn into fat.

SPICE UP YOUR LIFE!

It has long been known in cultures different from our own that herbs and spices can speed up fat burning. I think the flavours of garlic and chilli make vegetables much more exciting. Even though not all types of chillies are hot, I have experienced the burning tongue, the hot flushes and those pearls of sweat on the forehead. Different varieties of chillies and curry powders help to lift Indian and Mexican cuisine to new heights – and possibly make them burn more energy and fat, according to certain studies (Shahidi 2015, Yoshioka 1995, Ahuja 2006). The effects are modest, though, and the researchers have different explanations for the way it potentially works. It is known that a burning tongue activates a part of the nervous system that combats fat storage. The resulting waves of heat and hot flushes lead to a slightly higher energy burn.

Individual studies have shown that turmeric can slow down the storage of fat. It slows down the formation of blood vessels to the fat cells, so that it is more difficult for fat to take hold. Turmeric appears to increase insulin sensitivity so that glucose is more easily burned as energy instead of being stored as fat. Turmeric doesn't taste strong, so I sneak it into all the dinners I can. However, it does leave its mark in the form of persistent stains on clothes. I have sacrificed several shirts along the way, but with such a positive effect on health, maybe it was worth it.

Eastern spices can help to make losing weight a little easier – so don't leave your spices standing on the shelf. Spices with similar effects are chillies, cinnamon, cloves, black pepper and ginger (Aggarwal 2010). Spice up your life a bit more!

TIPS TO GET MORE SPICE IN YOUR DAILY LIFE

* Use turmeric in soups, casseroles and stir-fries.

* Make spicy Eastern-inspired dishes such as spicy lentil stew.

* Experiment with chilli in tomato sauces and soups.

* Sprinkle a little ground cinnamon over coffee with milk.

* Grind black pepper over evening meals and salads.

* Use fresh ginger in stir-fries, smoothies and dressings.

Now that you are standing on the threshold of the third of your 12 weeks to a slimmer waist, I like to think that you are already feeling the extra benefits and energy. Some of you will also feel happier and more motivated in your mind. Studies show that a diet based on pure ingredients, rather than refined and heavily processed food, has a significant effect on the mind and the rest of the body. While in the past you may have felt a bit trapped because of sugar cravings, and usually collapsed onto the sofa after dinner, now you are getting cravings for healthier flavours, and looking for challenges for which you used to lack energy. The steps you have taken up to now say it all about your future quality of life – the way ahead is exciting! In three weeks you have created habits that make life and your menu more colourful. Congratulate yourself with an experience or a little treat that your heart desires – you deserve it!

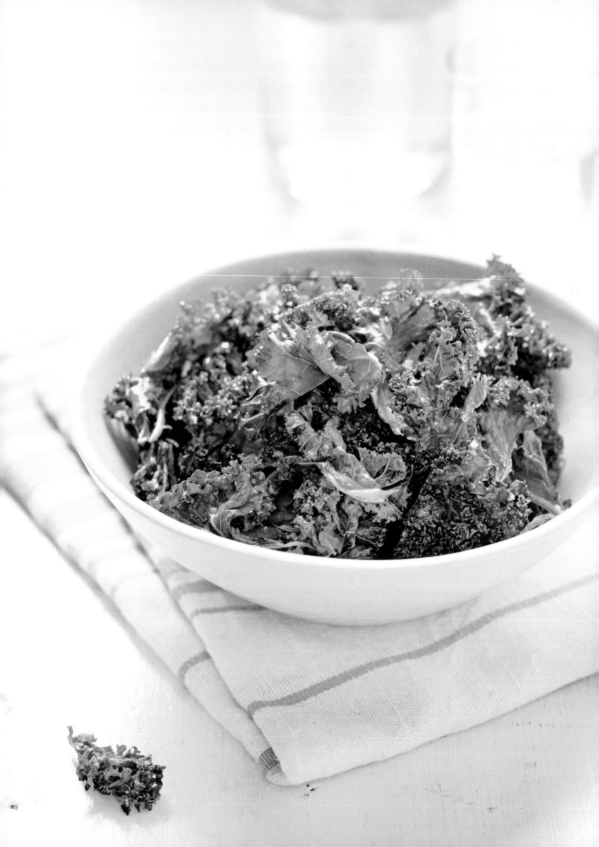

Kale chips, the world's healthiest snack

With kale you can make snacks that go down as well as potato chips.

3–4 kale leaves
2 tablespoons extra virgin olive oil
½ teaspoon sea salt (a good pinch)

Preheat the oven to 175°C (350°F).
Tear the kale leaves into pieces the size of potato chips and put them in a bowl. Add the olive oil and sea salt, and combine.
Spread the kale on a layer of baking paper on a baking tray.
Bake in the oven for 10–12 minutes. Take care that the kale doesn't turn brown or burn.

TIP: Make kale chips as a snack, or scatter them as a garnish over different evening meals such as pasta, fish dishes and salads. Vary the flavours by spicing up the kale with a little chilli or curry powder.

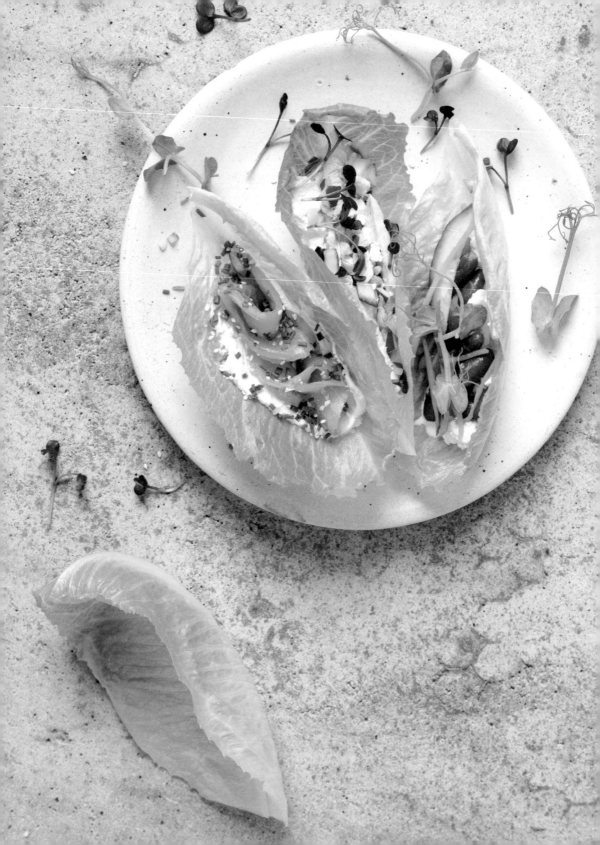

Green wraps

When you fill lettuce leaves with a little salmon, avocado, chives and a dash of sour cream, you get a great starter or snack. Play around with the ingredients in the list below.

WRAP:
Cos (romaine) lettuce

PROTEIN:
Tinned kidney beans (rinsed), cottage cheese, chicken or fish leftovers, egg, salmon, cheese, quinoa

CRISPY CRUNCHY VEGETABLES:
Grated carrot, cucumber, bean sprouts (trimmed), rocket (arugula), red onion (sliced)

SAUCE OR RELISH:
Nut butter, cream cheese, yoghurt, hummus, guacamole

SEEDS:
Pepitas (pumpkin seeds), sesame seeds, sunflower seeds

SAUCES, HERBS AND SPICES:
Tabasco, mustard, soy sauce, fish sauce, aioli, herbs, spices

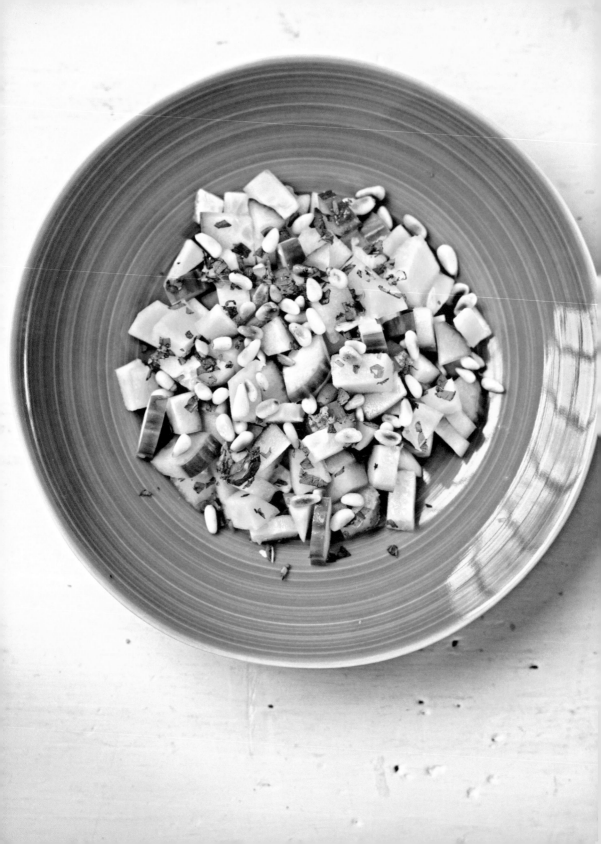

Cucumber and melon salad

This fresh, sweet and succulent salad is a summer favourite.

SERVES 4

1 rockmelon
1 cucumber
15–20 mint leaves
juice of 1 orange

Chop the rockmelon flesh and put it in a mixing bowl.
Chop the cucumber and mint leaves, and combine with the rockmelon. Add the orange juice
and mix well.
Place the cucumber and melon salad in a serving dish – then it's ready to enjoy!

TIPS: Add a few chopped nuts or crumbled feta cheese to the salad if you like. Fresh
blueberries also taste wonderful with it.

To create interesting serving dishes, you can use the melon shells. When preparing the salad,
cut the rockmelon in half and carefully cut out the flesh so that the melon shells become
two bowls. Place the melon shells on your serving dishes and spoon the salad inside.

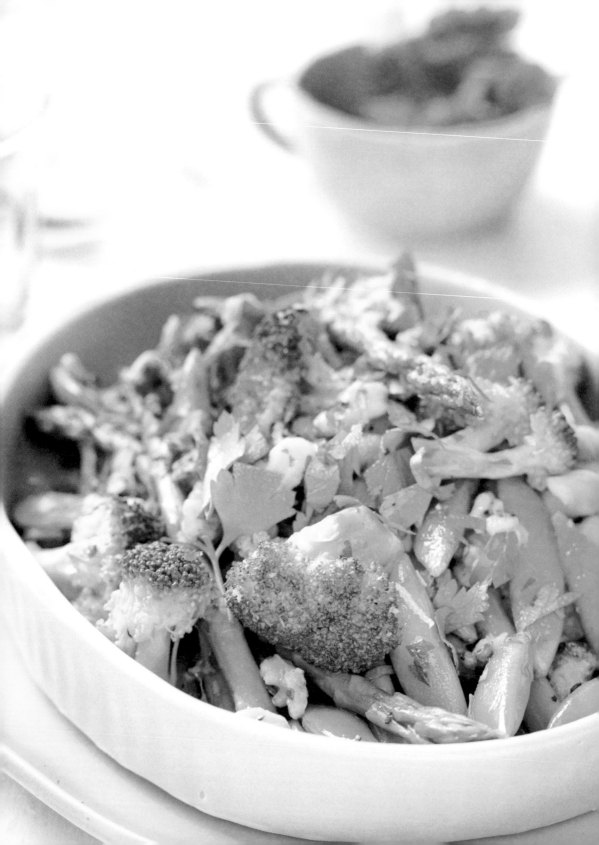

Gremolata

A dressing that is usually made of grated lemon zest, garlic, flat-leaf parsley and olive oil, gremolata is common in Italian cuisine and goes well with veal. Gremolata is super-quick to make and is splendid with blanched vegetables, such as green beans, broccoli florets, asparagus, or snap peas. Serve the vegetables as a stand-alone lunch dish with a little wholegrain bread, or on the side with meat or fish.

1
2
3
4

SERVES 4

450 g (1 lb) green vegetables, such as snap
  peas, broccoli florets or asparagus
sea salt and freshly ground black pepper

GREMOLATA

150 g (5½ oz) walnuts, chopped
4 tablespoons pine nuts
3 garlic cloves, chopped
1 tablespoon grated lemon zest
2 handfuls chopped flat-leaf (Italian) parsley
100 g (3½ oz) grated hard cheese,
  such as parmesan
90 ml (3 fl oz) extra virgin olive oil

Rinse the vegetables and cut them into small pieces.
Boil some water in a large saucepan. Put the vegetables into the boiling water, and blanch them for 2–3 minutes. Drain in a colander, then put them immediately in a bowl with ice cubes and water. That way they will keep their crispness and fresh green colour.
To make the gremolata, tip the walnuts and pine nuts into a dry frying pan. Cook them over low heat for 4–5 minutes.
Combine the garlic, lemon zest, parsley, parmesan and toasted nuts in a mixing bowl.
When you are ready to eat, heat the olive oil in a frying pan to a medium heat. Put the blanched vegetables in the pan, and lightly warm them for 2 minutes while stirring. Take the pan off the heat, and stir in the gremolata. Sprinkle over a little salt and pepper, and serve.

TIPS: Vary the recipe with different vegetables, and experiment with your own gremolata. Sage, mint and rosemary work well. Try other vegetables such as cauliflower florets or edamame (green soya beans). Use gremolata over steamed English spinach or grilled zucchini (courgette) and eggplant (aubergine) slices. The only limit is your imagination.

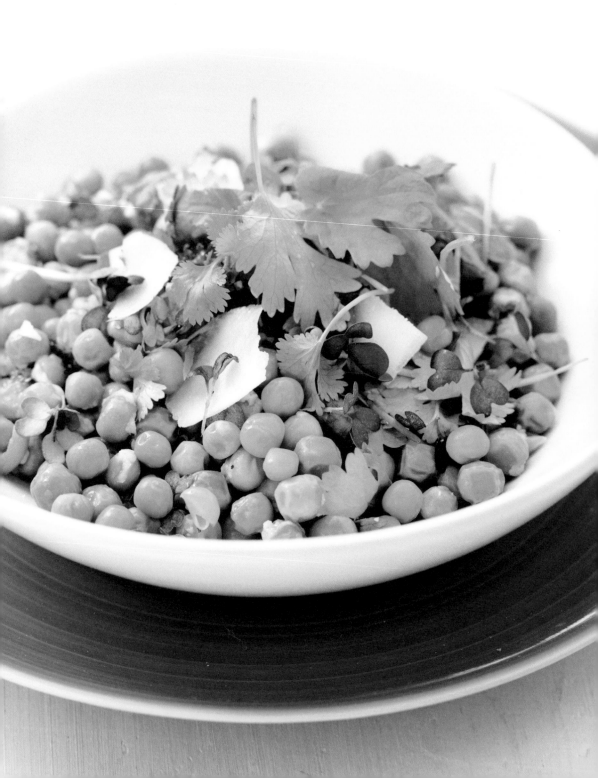

Tasty green peas

There's nothing simpler. Use the herbs you have in the kitchen –
I use flat-leaf parsley and coriander (cilantro). This dish is nice
as a side with meat or fish.

SERVES 4

350 g (12 oz) frozen green peas
1 tablespoon butter
1 large handful grated hard cheese, such as parmesan
2 handfuls fresh herbs
juice of ½ lemon and a little grated lemon zest
sea salt and freshly ground black pepper
parmesan cheese shavings

Boil the peas, then drain and rinse in a colander.
Put the peas back in the pan. Stir in the butter, grated cheese and fresh herbs.
Add the lemon juice, lemon zest, a pinch of sea salt and a little ground pepper to taste.
Serve with some parmesan shavings on top.

TIP: If you want, add other vegetables to the dish, such as chopped capsicum (pepper),
red onion or spring onions (scallions).

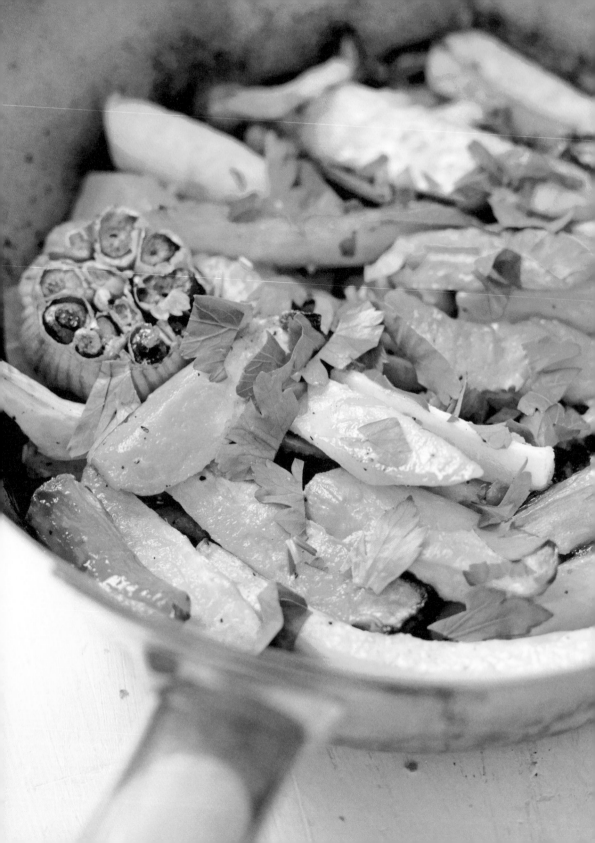

Root vegetables with parsley pesto

Parsley pesto gives sweet, oven-roasted root vegetables a lovely kick. Use the vegetables you have in the house, such as carrots, kohlrabi or parsnip. This dish is ideal with fish.

SERVES 4–5

600 g (1 lb 5 oz) root vegetables
3–4 tablespoons olive oil

PARSLEY PESTO
1 bunch flat-leaf (Italian) parsley, plus extra to garnish
50 g (1¾ oz) parmesan or other hard cheese
50 g (1¾ oz) toasted walnuts
2 garlic cloves
100 ml (3½ fl oz) extra virgin olive oil

Preheat the oven to 175°C (350°F).
Scrub or peel the vegetables, and cut into sticks. Bring a large saucepan of water to the boil, then add the vegetables and cook for 5–6 minutes.
Drain well, then transfer the vegetables to a roasting pan and drizzle the oil over. Roast for 40 minutes until they are tender and nicely coloured.
Blend the parsley, parmesan, walnuts, garlic and olive oil in a blender until you have a smooth parsley pesto.
Combine the root vegetables with the parsley pesto and set aside for 5 minutes before serving, so that the flavours can infuse.

TIP: If you like, add a whole garlic bulb to the roasting tin with the vegetables. Once cooked, pop the sweet flesh from the papery skins and mix through the finished dish.

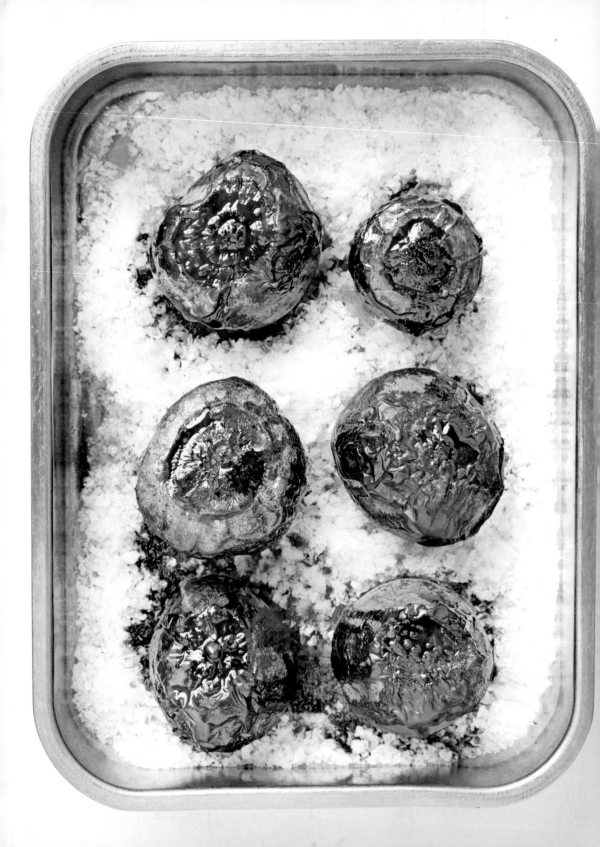

Salt-baked beetroot

Beetroot (beet) is a formidable source of plant energy, and develops a beautiful sweetness when baked in the oven.

8–10 small or 4–5 large beetroot (beets)
coarse rock salt or sea salt
extra virgin olive oil

Preheat the oven to 175°C (350°F).
Wash the beetroot, but don't peel them.
Fill an ovenproof dish with a layer of coarse salt, 5 mm–1 cm (¼–½ inch) thick. Push the beetroot down a little into the salt.
Drizzle with a little olive oil.
Bake the beetroot for 1½–2 hours, depending on their size, until they are tender.

TIP: Use this same recipe for whole onions, carrots and parsnips. If you like, you can combine several vegetables in the same dish. The vegetables can be served quite simply with a little butter and tarragon.

1

2

3

4

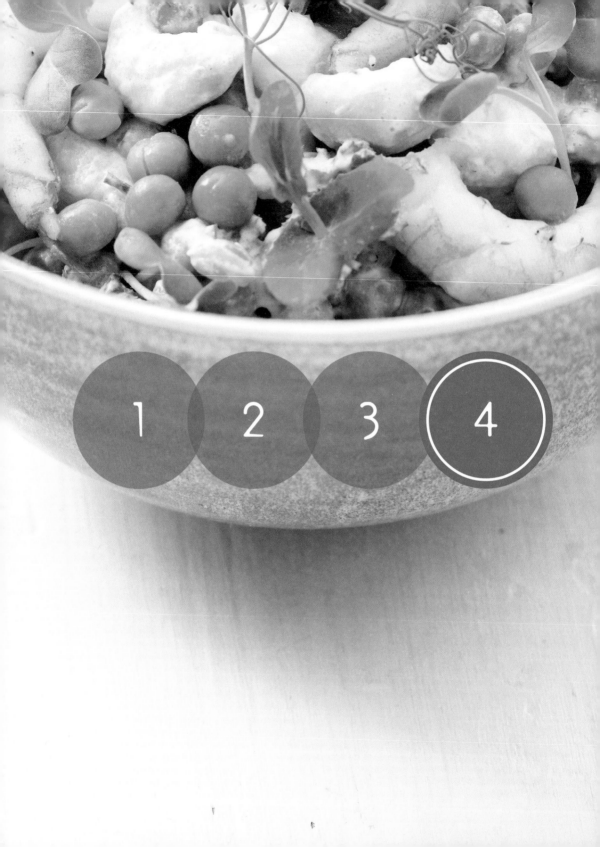

GOAL FOR WEEK 4

This week's exercise is to eat enough fish and seafood, and to cut out processed, hydrogenated fat from your daily meals. The Norwegian expression 'Eat fish to feel fresh' is embodied by consuming plenty of vitamin D, which increases fat burning, kills fat cells and builds muscle mass.

EAT FISH AND SEAFOOD WITH OMEGA-3 AND VITAMIN D

Now it has been three weeks, and you are well on the way. After last week's meal-enriching plant power, you have most likely begun to feel a bubbling energy. Take advantage of that energy and get out a little more, have fun with the kids or the grandkids, or start a walking group with friends. Perhaps you could invite some of them around for dinner in the middle of the week. If you don't feel any noticeable effect yet, this week's changes will do the trick: by eating enough fish, you'll get omega-3 and vitamin D into your daily diet. It's easier than you think!

Many people observe that they feel lighter after a meal of fish than after one of meat. But do you really lose weight by eating more fish? A lot of research indicates that the ocean's bounty can contribute in many ways, among others by increasing your burning of fat. Does that sound too good to be true? It isn't!

Oily fish provides a class of unsaturated fatty acids called omega-3. Plentiful supply of omega-3 strengthens a range of neurotransmitters and hormones in your body, insulin among them (Wallin 2012). Increased insulin sensitivity means that you don't have to make so much of it before your cells start burning blood sugar. You remember, of course, that big spikes in insulin lead to the storing of fat. Oilier fish therefore creates increased insulin sensitivity and results in better burning of fat. You'll find an abundance of omega-3 fatty acids in oily fish such as sardines, anchovies, herring, mackerel and salmon.

In the modern diet, a lot of omega-6 can easily curb the effect of omega-3. My son Petter notices the effect on his body when he eats junk food and ready-meals with fried fats and harmful plant oils. He can become unfocused and irritable, and is not willing to sacrifice his good mood to those tastes any more than once in a while. I make sure that he gets enough omega-3 in the form of capsules, and rejoice that we are able to balance his concentration and anxiety at a comfortable level in spite of his ADHD. Many studies show the benefits of more omega-3 in the diet. He is not so thrilled about spoonfuls of fish oil, so I am happy that there are capsules that slip down easily …

OILS THAT ARE RICH IN OMEGA-3 STAY FLUID, EVEN IN THE FRIDGE – IT'S LOGICAL, BECAUSE OTHERWISE OILY FISH WOULD BECOME RIGID IN THE COLD WATERS.

Limit omega-6 to strengthen omega-3

You need both omega-6 and omega-3 in your daily diet for your health to be at its best, but too much or too little can have adverse effects. The two fatty acids compete with each other in your body, so that too much omega-6 weakens the effect of omega-3. The modern diet is quickly becoming dominated by omega-6 fat from plant oils, margarine and ready-meals. Many of us now have 15–20 times more omega-6 in our diets than omega-3. The optimum ratio of omega-6 to omega-3 is 2:1. In this area, many of us have a long way to go. It's a good idea to avoid omega-6-rich plant oils such as corn oil, sunflower oil and soybean oil, and to choose more oily fish. Animals that chew grass and seeds have more omega-3 in their meat. Oily fish like herring, mackerel, anchovy and salmon contribute a lot of omega-3.

TIPS TO LIMIT YOUR INTAKE OF OMEGA-6

* Stop using omega-6 rich oils such as sunflower oil, corn oil and soybean oil.

* Avoid margarine – it's better to choose real butter.

* Avoid soy milk.

* Limit the use of processed food marked 'vegetable fat', because that is, as a rule, omega-6 oil.

Excess weight and bigger waist measurements also increase the risk of diabetes, cardiovascular disease and cancer. By looking after yourself with a little more fish, you can cut down blood pressure, reduce inflammation and reduce the level of oily acids that settle in the blood vessels. This protects you against the diseases already mentioned (He 2009, Lorente-Cebrián 2013). The omega-3 in fish will strengthen the effect of a range of neurotransmitters and hormones. That includes the fullness hormones, meaning that you feel full faster, so you eat less (Parra 2008). The proteins in fish also help your body to capture the omega-3.

Additionally, proteins delay the emptying of the stomach and make you feel pleasantly satisfied for longer. An increase in protein at your mealtimes can make it easier for you to maintain a stable ideal weight, even if the increase is modest. See page 156 to read more about how and why protein-rich ingredients can help you to reduce your waist size.

There is a sea of studies that point to the relationship between eating fish and seafood, and better health and a stronger mind. Gradually there have been more that claim that the ocean's bounty has a substantial influence on body weight. Several have made an impact: in one study, 324 overweight men and women were put into four groups that were followed for four weeks. The first group received sunflower oil capsules but no fish; the second group received three portions of lean fish – 150 g (5½ oz) firm white fish – per week; the third received three portions of oily fish – 150 g (5½ oz) salmon – per week; and the last group received fish oil but no fish. The calorific content of the groups' diets was exactly the same, but the diets with oily fish, lean fish and fish oil increased weight loss by an extra kilo in four weeks (Thorsdottir 2007). Many nutrients in fish make it easier for you to keep your weight down. If you can't get enough fish, take fish oil supplements – every little bit helps!

TIPS TO CONSUME MORE FISH PROTEIN

✳ Double the size of the pieces of fish that you serve – 150–175 g (5½–6 oz).

✳ Choose fish for dinner two or three times a week.

✳ Use fish leftovers in salads (I like smoked cod and salmon).

✳ Make sandwich toppings of fish, a little mayonnaise and fresh herbs.

Omega-3 and a good night's sleep

When you sleep badly, the fight against the kilos gets tougher. A series of studies has proven that there could be a relationship between a lack of sleep and weight gain. Fish can help here, too, because it has a sleep-inducing effect. Animal studies have shown that omega-3 fatty acids are great nutrients when your body produces hormones to improve sleep at night (Arias-Carrión 2011). Omega-3 and oily fish can actually lead to better quality sleep (Irmisch 2007). It's incredible what fish nutrients can help with – a flatter stomach, a clear mind, lower levels of tension, and a good night's sleep. Treat yourself to several fish dishes a week so that you never let this effect slip.

Sensible amounts of saturated fat

When it comes to saturated fat, there is not just one type. One study shows that if you replace some saturated fat from processed meat such as sausages, bacon and minced (ground) beef with pure fish and seafood, the burning of your subcutaneous fat increases and your waist size shrinks (Summers 2002).

TIPS ON HOW YOU CAN LIMIT YOUR INTAKE OF SATURATED FAT

* Replace sausage sandwiches with fish on flatbread.

* Make fish tacos instead of meat tacos.

* Replace meat sandwich toppings with fish toppings such as mackerel or herring.

* Replace paté with tuna.

* Replace bacon with trimmed, pan-fried prosciutto.

* Replace ice cream as a daily dessert with plain yoghurt, cottage cheese, vanilla extract and a little honey.

Cut out trans fats

Cut out all products with partially hydrogenated vegetable oils (also called trans fats), because they can increase the amount of belly fat. They can also increase your cholesterol to dangerous levels, create inflammation and contribute to obesity, insulin resistance, diabetes and metabolic syndrome (Micha 2009). As I always say, 'Hydrogenated fat gives food everlasting life … but puts you past your expiry date.'

A lot of trans fats have already been removed from ingredients and pre-prepared foods, but there is still a long way to go. A good tip is to avoid fried foods, and to check the ingredients in foods such as fatty snacks, cakes and biscuits. The best thing is to totally avoid such products.

GET YOUR VITAMIN D FROM BOTH OILY FISH AND SUPPLEMENTS

It has long been known that vitamin D increases mineral uptake and strengthens bone development, but it has even more important business than that. It helps the reading of genetic codes and ensures the efficient consumption and reproduction of neurotransmitters, hormones, muscle fibre and much more in your cells. Vitamin D is, somehow, the conductor of the orchestra of your cells. This vitamin creates more happiness hormones in your brain, so as I always say, 'When you're missing vitamin D, depression and dementia follow easily'. But is it a simple matter to fit a daily dose of vitamin D into your hectic life?

You can get enough vitamin D from oily fish, fish oil supplements, golden yellow egg yolks, and sunshine on your skin. It helps cells in your immune system to mature, divide and rebuild in order to strengthen your immunity – a defence that puts invaders like bacteria and viruses out of action while reducing inflammatory reactions in your body. A high level of inflammatory substances weakens the sensitivity of many neurotransmitters. When the amount of inflammatory substances is reduced, insulin sensitivity increases (page 23). When the insulin hormone is working better, it results in less insulin, less storing of fat and a slimmer waist.

Vitamin D takes the credit for an ever-increasing number of beneficial outcomes in the body. It can both increase fat burning and kill those cells when they are emptied of fat, so that the number of fat cells actually diminishes (Sergeev 2009). This mechanism is logical in the animal kingdom, because a lower level of vitamin D during the colder, darker times of the year means that fat burning is reduced while fat is stored. That keeps animals warmer. When the sun warms up again, vitamin D production in the skin increases, fat burning gains momentum and subcutaneous fat is burned off. Sunlight, sunny egg yolks, oily fish and offal can all trigger this mechanism.

When I was studying medicine in the 1980s, we learned this formula: calories in > calories out = weight gain. Now we know that weight is a function of both calories and the nutrients that program your body's cells. Food is much more than just energy!

A study of 102 Spanish schoolchildren demonstrated a relationship between low levels of vitamin D, high BMI and a high proportion of body fat (Rodríguez-Rodríguez 2010).

A little more fish on your plate helps you to burn fat and build muscle mass. That is because your muscle cells then secure enough vitamin D conductors to produce muscle protein effectively. While having only a small number of conductors leads to fat being stored inside the muscle cells, a sufficient amount of vitamin D results in fat being replaced by strong muscle fibre (Gilsanz 2010). You can reprogram your body, from fat storing and weakened muscles, to fat burning and increased muscle power with the help of delicious fish dishes!

Should you take omega-3 and vitamin D supplements?

Omega-3 uptake from the dinner plate varies from person to person, and too many of us eat too little fish to ensure that we get a sufficient amount. The production of vitamins in the skin declines with age, so depending on the amount of sunlight you are exposed to, you might need to take a supplement. Not all countries have expressed an opinion on what ought to be the upper limit for omega-3 consumption. While the US Food and Drug Administration has previously concluded that it is safe to take up to 3 g (⅒ oz) per day of marine omega-3 fatty acids (Kris-Etherton 2002), the European Food Safety Authority (EFSA) has now raised the upper limit for consumption to 5 g (⅙ oz) (EFSA 2012). The consumption of 2–4 g (¼₁₄–⅐ oz) of omega-3 daily is what you should aim for in order to reduce blood pressure and the amount of damaging fat (triglycerides) in the blood. If you feel that you need a higher dose, you shouldn't increase the amount of fish oil by too many tablespoons. That can lead to a high intake of vitamin A, so it's better to buy high-dosage capsules with omega-3.

Do you avoid fish oil supplements because of an allergy? You may not need to – many products are free from the fish proteins that trigger allergies. Vitamin D supplements can be beneficial if we suffer a lack of vitamin D during the winter months (Norkost 3). So, choose an omega-3 supplement with added vitamin D and measure your vitamin D level to see if it is high enough.

Delicious fish provides a lot of muscle mass per calorie, making it easier to learn and to remember, lifting the mood, and giving better weight control and a long-lasting sensation of fullness. Blood pressure drops, inflammation is kept in check and the immune system is strengthened. Let the trip to the fish market become a part of your daily routine.

GREAT ADVICE FOR CONSUMING MORE FISH EVERY DAY

* Search online for fish dishes and pick out two easy recipes every week.

* Vary between oily and lean fish.

* Replace the meat with fish in some traditional dishes, such as salads, casseroles and stir-fries.

* Make salad and sandwich toppings with fish (see pages 97 and 99).

* If you work in a place with a canteen, ask if they can make more fish dishes.

* Buy fish at a fish market or at a shop with a fish counter.

* Go fishing yourself.

GREAT ADVICE FOR ACHIEVING BETTER OMEGA-3 RESULTS FOR YOUR BODY

* Take fish oil or capsules with vitamin D.

* Eat omega-3 rich nuts and seeds such as walnuts, pecans, crushed linseeds (flaxseeds) or chia seeds. For example, when serving rolled (porridge) oats, stir in a few chopped nuts and seeds, or add a few to smoothies and yoghurts.

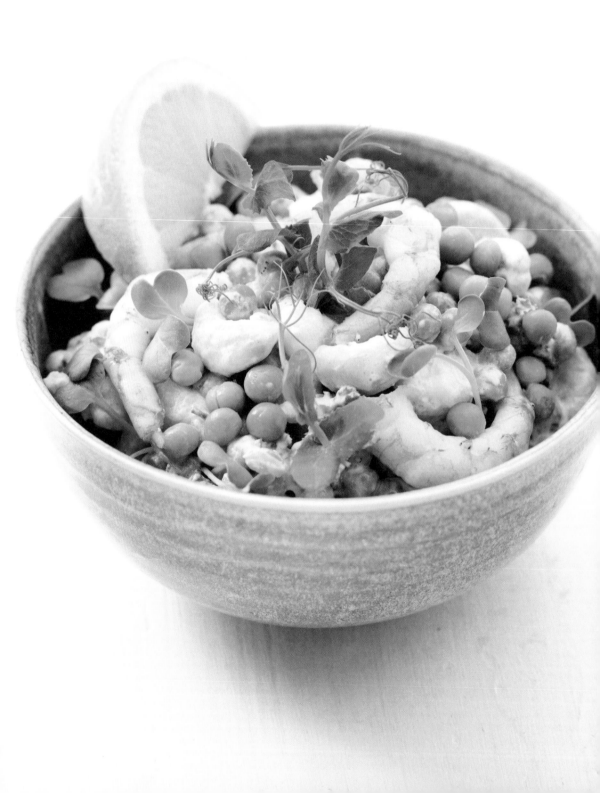

Pea salad with prawns and cashew nuts

You can make this brilliant salad in just a few minutes, and it tastes really good. Try it for lunch.

SERVES 4

30 g (1 oz) sour cream
30 g (1 oz) plain yoghurt
1 big squeeze of lemon juice
2 teaspoons chopped fresh chives
fresh dill, flat-leaf (Italian) parsley or other herbs (optional)
freshly ground black pepper
250 g (9 oz) cooked peeled prawns (shrimp)
250 g (9 oz) frozen peas, thawed and drained
100 g (3½ oz) roasted unsalted cashew nuts

Make a dressing by mixing together the sour cream, yoghurt, lemon juice, chives, herbs and pepper.
Rinse the prawns in a little cold water.
Stir the prawns and the peas into the dressing until well combined.
Scatter over the cashew nuts just before serving. If you do this too far in advance, the nuts will soak up the dressing.

TIP: The quality of the yoghurt and sour cream that you use will have a big effect on the result. The salad can be served with a handful of mild salad leaves, such as baby English spinach, if you like.

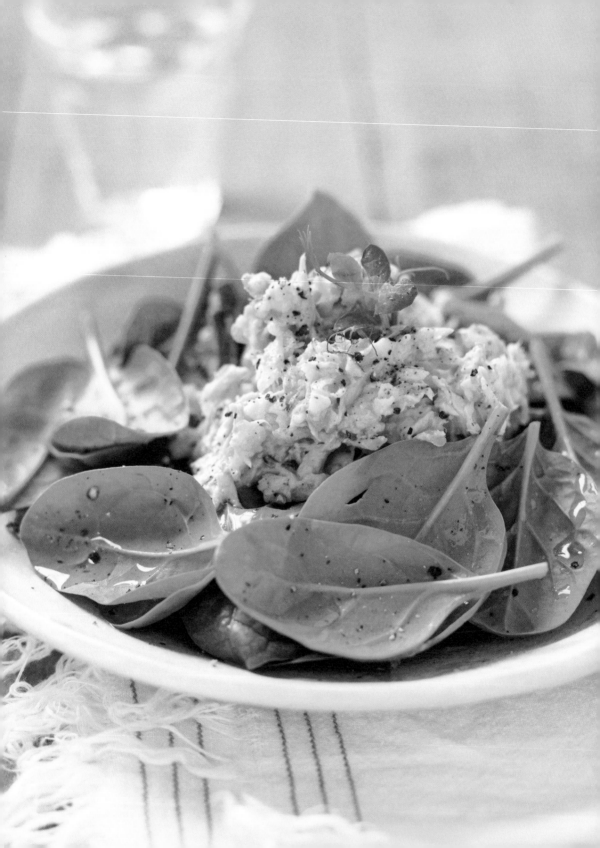

Salmon salad

You can have a fish salad for lunch or for dinner, or as topping on a slice of bread for breakfast.

SERVES 2

300 g (10½ oz) pre-cooked or steamed salmon
2 large carrots
1 apple
1 tablespoon of your favourite mustard
2 tablespoons extra virgin olive oil
2 heaped tablespoons mayonnaise
juice of ½ lemon
sea salt and freshly ground black pepper
fresh herbs (optional)

Cut the salmon into pieces.
Peel and grate the carrots. Grate the apple with the peel on.
Put all the ingredients in a bowl and mix well with a fork.

SERVING TIP: Lay a good portion of salmon salad on a bed of two handfuls of baby English spinach. Scatter over some roasted pine nuts and serve with a slice of fresh bread – then you'll have a lunch for even the most demanding guests.

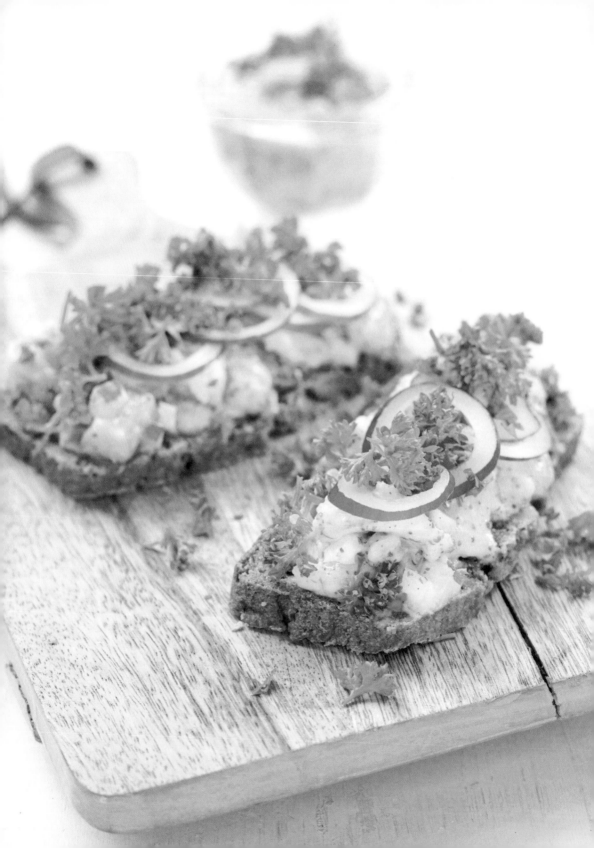

Mustard herring

Mustard herring is simple to make at home. It only demands that you start a couple of days before you wish to eat it. It's a super way to enjoy small amounts of omega-3-rich fish in your daily life – the whole year round.

SERVES 4

4 salted or pickled herring fillets
½ red onion
1 large bunch fresh dill
100 g (3½ oz) mayonnaise, sour cream or crème fraîche
1–2 tablespoons of your favourite mustard, or a mix of dijon and regular mustard
1 teaspoon apple cider vinegar, white wine vinegar, or another vinegar of your choice
2 teaspoons honey

First, if using salted herring, you must draw out the salt. This is easily done, by soaking the fillets in water overnight, preferably for 24 hours. Always taste a little bit before you mix the herring and the sauce! If the herring is too salty, let it soak again for another night.
Finely chop the red onion and the dill.
Blend the dill, red onion, mayonnaise, mustard, vinegar and honey into a sauce.
Cut the herring fillets into small pieces and lay them on a large plate in layers with the sauce in between.
Leave the herring in the fridge for at least 1 day.

SERVING TIP: This tastes great served on seeded bread, scattered with flat-leaf parsley and onion slices and garnished with freshly ground black pepper or curry powder (optional).

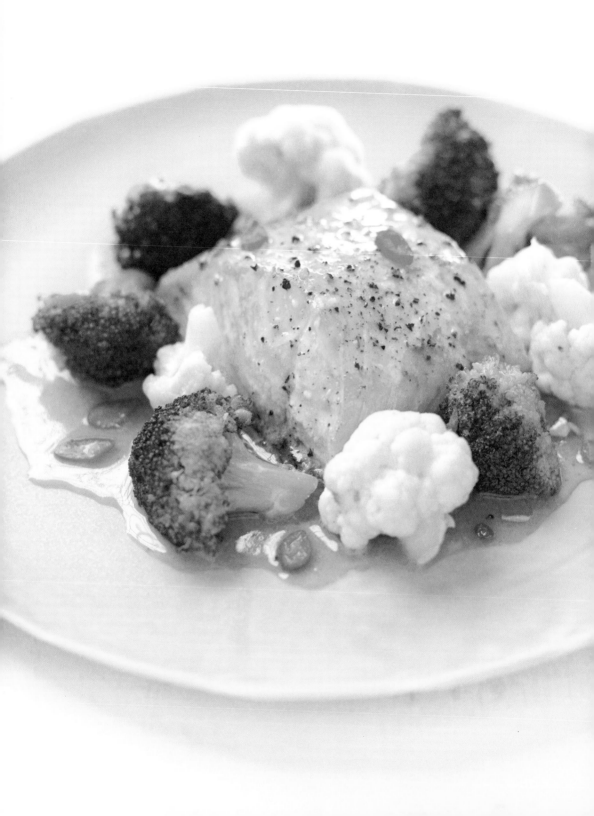

Nice and easy salmon dinner

This is a twist on a recipe I made on the Norwegian TV show *Schrödinger's Cat*, when I had to demonstrate that it was possible for a student to make an entire tasty, fully nutritious meal in the same time it took to bake a frozen pizza.

SERVES 1

300 g (10½ oz) vegetables, for example a frozen mixed bag, or 100 g (3½ oz) broccoli, 100 g (3½ oz) cauliflower and 100 g (3½ oz) carrots
2–3 garlic cloves
1 tablespoon butter, for frying
120–150 g (4¼–5½ oz) salmon fillet
sea salt and freshly ground black pepper
2 tablespoons sour cream
1 tablespoon soy sauce
1 teaspoon honey
a little sweet chilli sauce

Preheat the oven to 200°C (400°F).
If you are using fresh vegetables, cut the broccoli and cauliflower into florets, and the carrot into slices.
Chop the garlic. Melt the butter in a frying pan, and add all the vegetables. Let them sauté until tender while you prepare the salmon.
Season the salmon with salt and pepper. Cook it for 12–15 minutes in the oven.
Stir together the sour cream, soy sauce, honey and sweet chilli sauce, and pour over the salmon for the last 5 minutes of cooking.
Place the cooked vegetables on a plate. Put the salmon on top, dribbling the sour cream sauce over to finish.

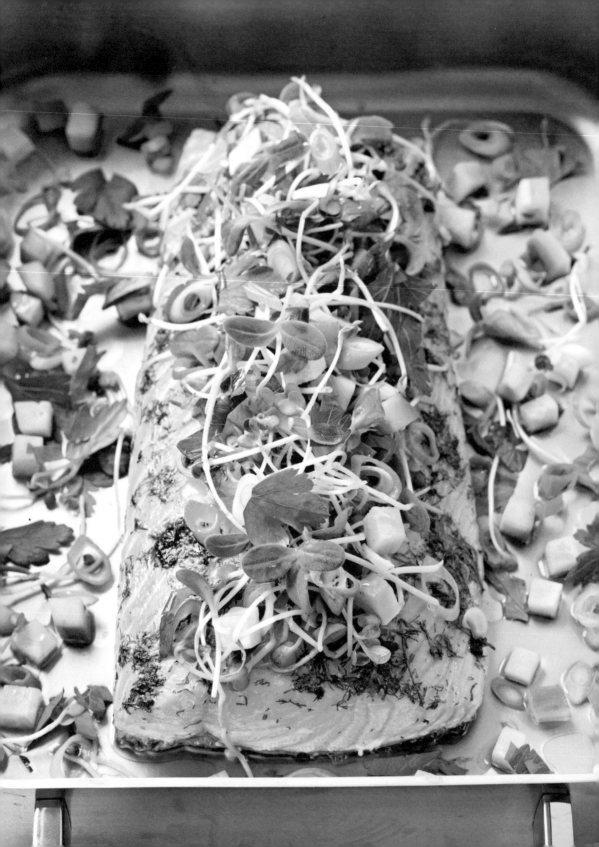

Oven-roasted salmon with dill

This is probably my children's favourite recipe, especially when the salmon is served with pearl barley and a dollop of sour cream. You can use any leftovers in the salmon salad on page 97. Fresh dill tastes best in this dish, but dried dill is also good.

SERVES 4–5

extra virgin olive oil
800 g–1 kg (1 lb 12 oz–2 lb 4 oz) piece salmon with skin
sea salt
lots of fresh or dried dill
finely diced cucumber, chopped spring onion (scallion), flat-leaf parsley and microherbs,
  to garnish

Preheat the oven to 160°C (315°F).
Brush an ovenproof dish with a little olive oil. Put the salmon in the dish with the skin side down. Brush the salmon with olive oil.
Sprinkle a little sea salt over the fish, followed by lots of dill. The fish should be completely green on top.
Cook the fish in the oven for about 20 minutes, until it is just light pink and firm to the touch when you press down with a fork.

TIP: Roast a little broccoli along with the salmon, and cook up some pearl barley instead of white rice. Mix different types of lettuce in a big bowl, and voilà – you've got a complete dinner, ready to go.

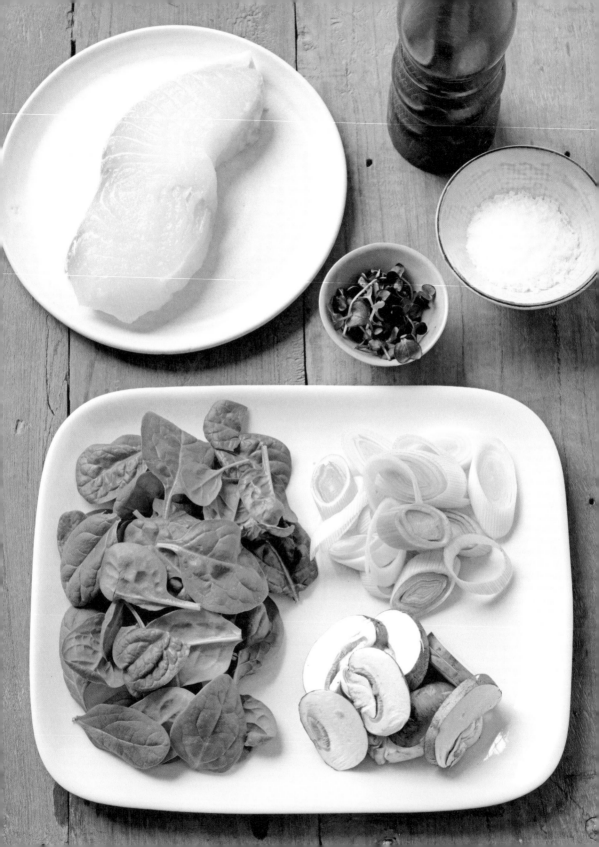

Steamed fish

Steamed white fish is excellent fast food if you have no idea what to make for dinner or if you are in a rush. The really clever thing with this nutritious dish is that you can steam all the ingredients at the same time, so this great tasting dinner is ready in only 10 minutes. A simple dressing with ginger, garlic and chilli gives it a lovely touch and a lot of antioxidants that both strengthen the immune system and curb inflammatory disorders in the body.

SERVES 4

sea salt and freshly ground black pepper
4 fillets firm white-fleshed fish, about
   125–150 g (4½–5½ oz) per piece
1 leek, white part only
around 12 fresh shiitake mushrooms,
   chestnut mushrooms or other mushrooms
200 g (7 oz) baby English spinach

DRESSING
1–2 garlic cloves, crushed
1 tablespoon grated fresh ginger
3 tablespoons freshly squeezed lemon juice
   or 1 tablespoon grated lemon zest
1 tablespoon soy sauce
1 tablespoon extra virgin olive oil
freshly ground black pepper (optional)

Mix all the ingredients for the dressing in a bowl, and set aside.
Sprinkle a little salt and pepper over the fish fillets. Fill the base of a steamer with water. Make sure there is plenty of space between the water and the base of the steaming basket. Bring the water to a simmer and then remove from the heat.
Cut the leek into 5 mm (¼ inch) thick rings and the mushrooms into 5 mm (¼ inch) thick slices. Place the leek in the steaming basket. Be careful that the steam doesn't burn you! Top with the mushroom pieces, and finally the fish fillets. Put the lid on, place the pan back on the heat, and let it steam for 3 minutes.
Take the pan off the heat and carefully lift the lid. You should be able to see that the fish has begun to change colour and texture. Sprinkle over the baby English spinach, put the pan back on the heat and let it steam for around 6 minutes, until the fish is firm and juicy.
Lay the fish on a bed of spinach, leek and mushroom, and drizzle a spoonful of dressing over each piece of fish before serving. If you like, serve with pearl barley, burghul (bulgur) or quinoa.

TIP: If you don't have a steamer, you can use a colander over a metal saucepan.

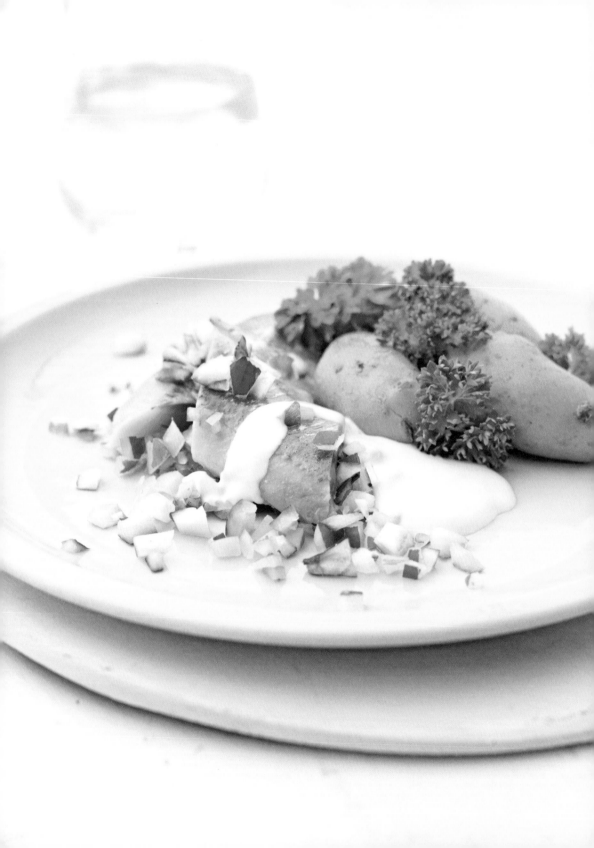

Spiced herring for dinner

SERVES 3–4

6–8 vacuum-packed spiced herring fillets (or pickled herring)
3–4 tablespoons chopped red onion
1 handful fresh flat-leaf (Italian) parsley
2–3 boiled new potatoes per person
1 tablespoon sour cream per person
green salad, to serve
crackers, to serve

Dish the herring out on a plate and scatter over the red onion and parsley.
Serve the herring with boiled new potatoes, a dollop of sour cream, plenty of green salad
and a few crackers.

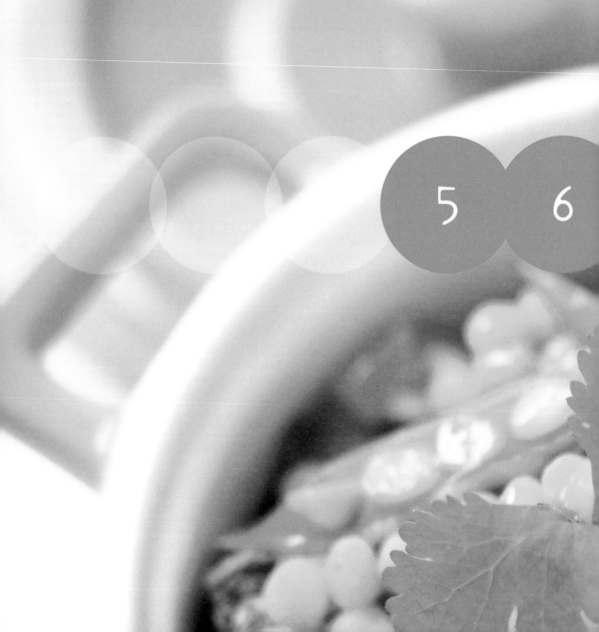

WEEKS 5–8

5 6

The next four weeks of this program pursue effective changes in diet that really contribute to shrinking the waist. With more fish and seafood, ingredients that strengthen the environment for bacteria, varied sources of protein and the right kind of fat, you can look forward to a slimmer body, improved memory and a stronger mind.

7 8

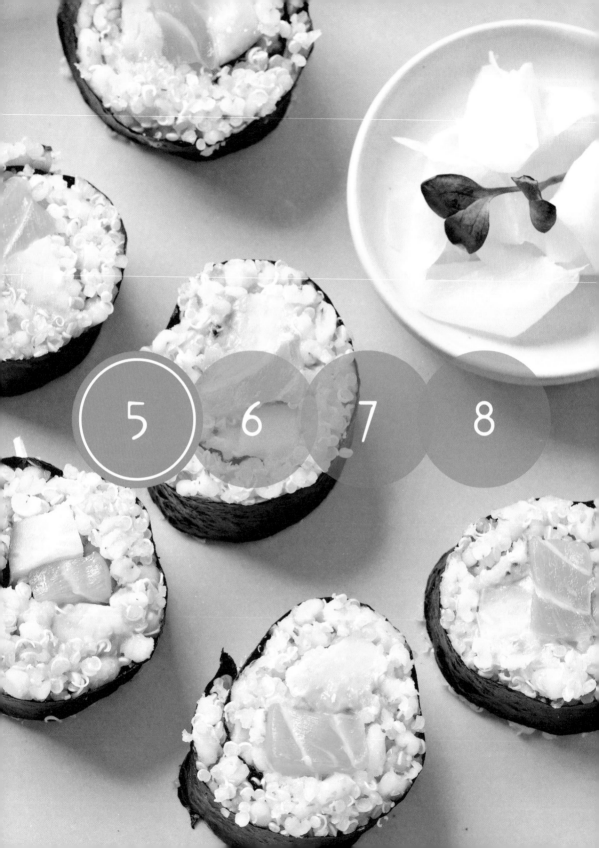

5 6 7 8

GOAL FOR WEEK 5

This week's exercise is to replace white rice and pasta with nutritious alternatives. You will experience how smart rice substitutes stabilise blood sugar levels, give you more energy, improve mood and eliminate troublesome cravings. And if the waist shrinks, too? Just see it as an added bonus.

EAT LENTILS, PEARL BARLEY AND QUINOA

THE WORD 'REFINED' SOUNDS SO GOOD. IT SUGGESTS SOMETHING GENTLY FORMED, SOMETHING HIGHLY CULTURED, EVEN. I LIKE PEOPLE WITH REFINED MINDS, BUT WHEN IT COMES TO FOOD, REFINEMENT USUALLY LEADS TO UNFORTUNATE CONSEQUENCES FOR BOTH QUALITY AND NUTRITIOUS CONTENT. IN THIS CONTEXT, REFINING ACTUALLY IMPLIES THE STRIPPING AWAY OF USEFUL NUTRIENTS. THE RESULT IS WHITE RICE, WHITE SUGAR AND WHITE WHEAT – A COLOUR THAT IS 'CLEAN' IN THE SENSE THAT IT IS CLEAN OF VITAMINS, FIBRE, PLANT NUTRIENTS AND A RANGE OF MINERALS!

THE REFINING OF RICE AND WHEAT MEANS THAT THE OUTER LAYERS OF THE RICE AND THE GRAIN ARE REMOVED SO THAT YOU ARE LEFT WITH ONLY THE STARCH-HEAVY CORE. BOTH BRAN AND WHEAT GERM, TWO IMPORTANT COMPONENTS OF THE CORE, ARE LOST. THAT'S UNFORTUNATE BECAUSE FIBRE, VITAMINS, MINERALS, AMINO ACIDS, FATTY ACIDS AND A RANGE OF PLANT NUTRIENTS ALSO VANISH. THE MOST NUTRITIOUS PARTS ARE THEREFORE REMOVED DURING REFINING.

WHEAT SEEMS TO BE PARTICULARLY UNLUCKY, BECAUSE MODERN WHEAT HAS MUCH STRONGER STARCH THAN BEFORE. SUCH 'SUPER-STARCH' MEANS A MUCH BIGGER SUGAR LOAD ON YOUR BODY, COMPARED TO ANCIENT VARIETIES OF WHEAT LIKE EINKORN OR EMMER. SPELT CAN BE BETTER THAN MODERN WHEAT, BUT YOU SHOULD CHOOSE A MORE OLD-WORLD SPELT. I LIKE TO CHOOSE ORGANIC SPELT IN ORDER TO GET AN ORIGINAL VARIETY RATHER THAN A HYBRID THAT IS CROSSED WITH MODERN WHEAT. THERE IS SUPER-STARCH IN BOTH WHOLEMEAL (WHOLE-WHEAT) AND REFINED WHEAT FLOUR. IT'S NO LONGER JUST BEER THAT HAS AN IMPACT ON THE WAIST IN THE FORM OF A BEER BELLY – WHEAT BELLY HAS BECOME A NEW CONCEPT, TOO.

SHARP SPIKES IN BLOOD SUGAR CREATE BELLY FAT

When fibre and plant nutrients are removed from foods, bacteria in the intestine no longer needs to break the food down before it is absorbed in smaller pieces in the gut. The digestive enzymes are released so easily that sugar chains are broken up into small compounds that are absorbed at the speed of lightning. Refined rice and pasta made with modern wheat provide masses of these carbohydrates that are devoured in a flash in the gut. That triggers the blood sugar alarm that chases down stress hormones round your body, setting off sky-high spikes in insulin and leading to the storing of fat around the waist.

The glucose causes proteins that are carried in the bloodstream to become sticky. They change characteristics – just like a woolly sock gets stuck to a puddle of soft drink spilled on the floor, they get stuck to a little bit of everything. It can increase your susceptibility to type-2 diabetes, high blood pressure, cardiovascular disease, metabolic syndrome and cancer. Read more about how steep spikes in blood sugar levels can create a heavy burden on page 49 (Week 2).

Fluctuating blood sugar and sky-high insulin spikes gradually deaden the 'insulin locks' in your cells. Then you'll need more 'insulin keys' for the cells to open the doors and let glucose in. There is a limit to how many keys your pancreas can produce. When your demand for these keys is no longer met, the cells struggle to allow glucose in for burning, leading to insulin resistance. If you continue to eat fast carbohydrates, they will therefore challenge more of your body's organ systems – not just your waist measurement.

5

6

7

8

Modern wheat and increasing occurrence of food intolerance and coeliac disease

Modern wheat is a totally different grain than that which your great-grandmother used to bake with. Modern wheat has more of one type of strong gluten than many can tolerate. When the wheat comes with both super-gluten and super-starch, the bread can rise up to high heaven. However, many of us have bacterial flora in the intestine that is not used to breaking down the masses of super-gluten we consume. That can create gluten intolerance disorders such as stomach pains, flatulence and diarrhoea. Modern super-gluten can also trigger gluten allergies, also called coeliac disease, among people with a genetic predisposition to it (van den Broeck 2010). Modern wheat and gluten-enriched products share part of the blame for the increasing occurrence of coeliac disease today. In Finland, for example, the prevalence has doubled in the last 20 years (Lohi 2007).

Inflammation is normally a tool that the body uses to keep itself healthy. It is the result of an immune system activated against invaders like bacteria and viruses, or against damaged tissue cells that need to be swept away – for example, during muscle fibre rupture. Your immune system, however, can also be triggered by refined or processed food. Additives and heavy processing change ingredients so that your immune system no longer recognises the food as 'natural'. The immune system gears up for the fight and produces an immune reaction as a weapon. The result can be that you end up with a high level of irritating inflammatory substances in your whole body.

Modern gluten weakens the bacterial flora and increases the amount of inflammatory substance in your body. That can harm the intestinal mucosa so that the contaminants, which a healthy mucosa would normally reject, are allowed to pass through. These contaminants alert the immune system to prepare for battle, depending on what your immune system perceives as a contaminant. You may experience symptoms such as headaches, nausea, joint and muscle pains, mental health disorders and low energy. You ought to get rid of this millstone when you want to lose weight, that's for sure!

GREAT ADVICE FOR CONSUMING LESS GLUTEN IN DAILY LIFE

* Choose old wheat varieties when you bake everyday bread.

* Limit the amount of pasta in your diet and replace it with salad or vegetables.

* Swap pasta for quinoa, lentils and/or barley.

* Replace burghul (bulgur) and couscous with beans or greens.

* Make vegetable noodles (see page 119).

Fat around your belly can actually create inflammatory substances all on its own. These are called cytokines, and add more weight to the burden of inflammation (Ouchi 2011). The greater the belly fat, the greater the disruption from inflammatory substances in many types of cells in the liver, muscles, other fat tissue, the pancreas, heart and brain.

Did you know that 40% of your belly fat is inflammatory cells, and that these, together with the belly fat cells, churn out irritating inflammatory substances all day long?

An increased level of inflammatory substances in the blood is connected to obesity, type-2 diabetes, cardiovascular disease, stroke, cancer, asthma, chronic bronchitis, swelling of the muscles and joints, depression disorders and dementia (Osborn 2012).

These inflammatory substances can also graze the blood vessel walls and make it easier for cholesterol to clog them up. In large population studies, increased occurrences of cardiovascular disease have been seen among those who are gluten intolerant (Ludvigsson 2009).

5

6

7

8

INCREASED APPETITE AND CRAVINGS

Gluten, milk and soy can create cravings, something that some scientists believe is due to the small amounts of protein that occur in the digestion of those foods. The theory assumes that such proteins act on the same 'door locks' as endorphins do (Teschemacher 2003), which can trigger addiction and dependence. Many people actually experience withdrawal symptoms, such as low energy levels, muddled thinking, irritability and depression when they stop consuming wheat products. There are many similarities, therefore, between addiction and bingeing on refined carbohydrates (Ifland 2009). Refined carbohydrates barely give a moment's pleasure before they toss out another nagging thought, pulling you into a vicious circle where wheat and sugar prompt cravings for more of the same … The addict stumbles ever more into incidents of addiction, satisfying big and small cravings alike with buns and biscuits, or with gallons of milk and ice cream. One of my patients could stand in front of the fridge door and drink the milk carton dry – a dependency that triggered anger, anxiety and poor concentration.

Sweetness and starch live in fruit, berries, wild rice and whole grains, along with fibre, water, vitamins, minerals and plant nutrients. Just like the instruments in an orchestra can, together, create a beautiful symphony, the differing nutrients in whole rice and whole grains compose a coherent 'song' that the body can use to a greater degree than each individual instrument. When rice and wheat are refined, they lose nutrients, and so the effects they have on the body are radically changed.

To break the cycle you will now replace white rice and pasta with whole grain rice or wild rice (nutrient-rich, unpolished rice grain, just as nature created) and naturally gluten-free grain and gluten-free seeds. But be careful with products labelled 'gluten free'! Many products that are marked 'gluten free' – especially ready-meals – are full of cornflour (cornstarch) that turns your blood sugar into syrup. Such products are, therefore, not healthy.

GREAT REPLACEMENTS FOR WHITE RICE AND PASTA

* Brown rice, wild rice

* Buckwheat

* Quinoa

* Barley

* Peas, beans and lentils

* Small chopped or shredded vegetables such as carrots, cauliflower or zucchini (courgettes)

Think outside the box. Who says that it has to be white rice that accompanies the casserole? Or traditional pasta with spaghetti bolognese? But don't stay away from all carbohydrates – your body needs them. Over the last hundred years we have fallen in love with the wrong type of carbohydrates. We need to replace the fast, refined, white ones that are everywhere these days.

Combined with good sources of protein and natural fats, slow carbohydrates contribute to better energy, good intestinal functioning, lower anxiety, improved sleep, long-lasting fullness and a stable ideal weight. Enjoy them in their natural wholeness, not as refined parts!

HOW TO COOK BROWN RICE

I always rinse rice, lentils and beans in cold water before I cook them. Rinse well, preferably several times, until the water runs clear. This removes the excess starch that is found on the outside of the grains and also all the dust that has gone into the packet with the grains. Additionally, rinsing prevents the rice grains from sticking together during cooking. In the pan, I use two parts water to one part rice. Bring the rice to the boil, before turning down the heat and letting it simmer for about 45 minutes. If you soak the rice overnight, the cooking time is shorter. Most whole grains (for example, barley) can be cooked in the same way as rice.

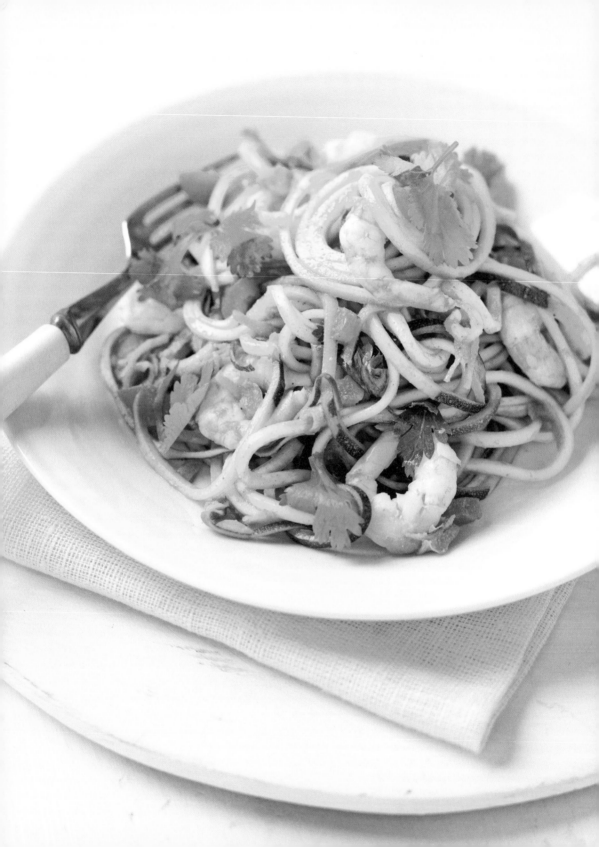

Stir-fried zucchini noodles

Pasta doesn't need to be made from wheat flour. You can just as easily make noodles from root vegetables, zucchini (courgettes) or broccoli stalks.

SERVES 4

2 zucchini (courgettes)
1 red capsicum (pepper)
3 garlic cloves
2 carrots
coconut oil, for frying
2 teaspoons grated fresh ginger
150 g (5½ oz) peeled raw prawns (shrimp) or other source of protein that
  you fancy, or leftovers
1 tablespoon curry powder
juice of 1 lime
2 teaspoons fish sauce
3 teaspoons sesame oil
freshly ground black pepper
2 handfuls chopped coriander (cilantro) leaves

Make the zucchini noodles with a spiralizer. Chop the capsicum and the garlic. Grate the carrots. Heat the coconut oil in a wok over medium heat, add the garlic and ginger and cook for 1 minute. Add the capsicum and let it sauté for 1 minute before you add the grated carrot, then sauté for a further minute.
Add the prawns, curry powder and zucchini noodles, and sauté for 1–2 minutes until the prawns are cooked through.
Stir through the lime juice, fish sauce, sesame oil, pepper and coriander leaves, and serve.

SERVING TIP: Place in a bowl and scatter with your usual nuts and seeds.

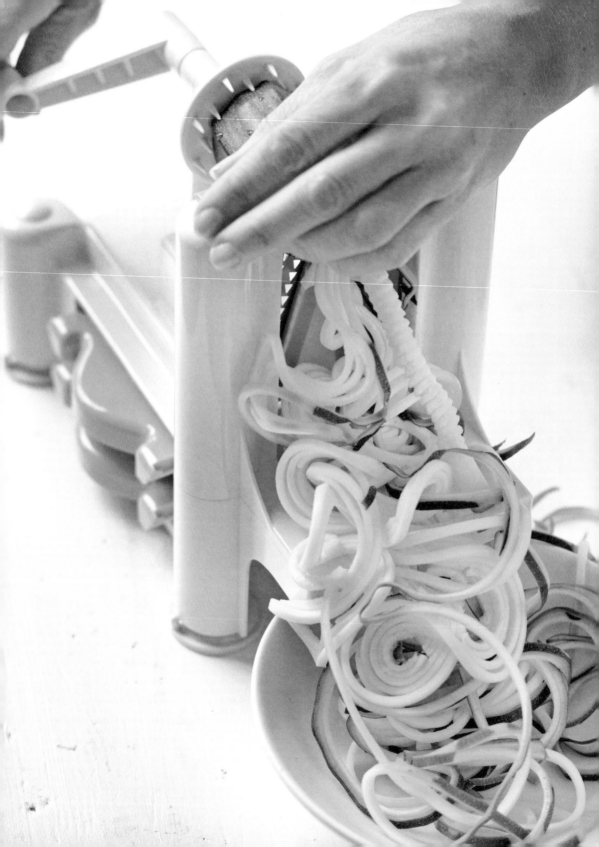

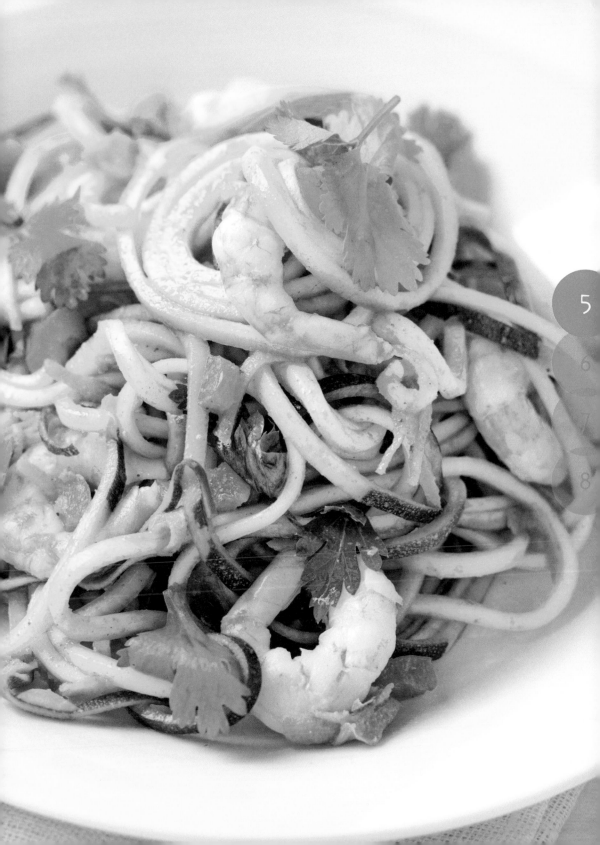

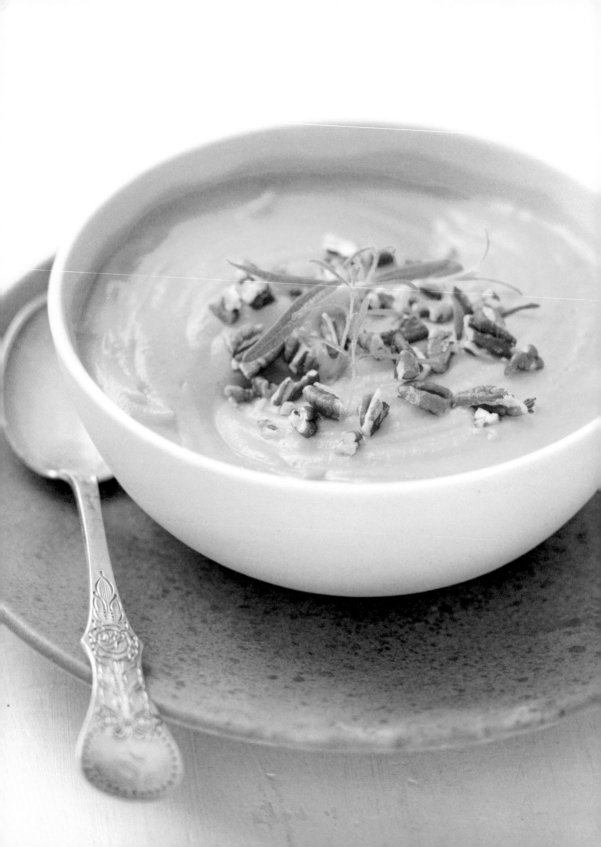

Sweet potato mash

This simple, antioxidant-rich, sweet potato mash tastes really good with both meat and chicken dishes.

SERVES 4–6

3–4 sweet potatoes, about 800 g (1 lb 12 oz)
200 ml (7 fl oz) milk
1 tablespoon butter
a little sea salt

Steam the sweet potatoes for around 45 minutes until they are tender and the skins begin to loosen slightly. Let them cool down a little.
Remove the sweet potato skins. It's easy when they are cooked – you can almost tear them off. Put the sweet potatoes, milk, butter and salt in a bowl. Blend with a stick blender to a smooth and even consistency.

TIP: Put the finished sweet potato mash in an ovenproof dish, sprinkle over chopped pecans and heat the mash in the oven at 160°C (315°F) just before serving. Be careful that the pecans don't burn.

5

6

7

8

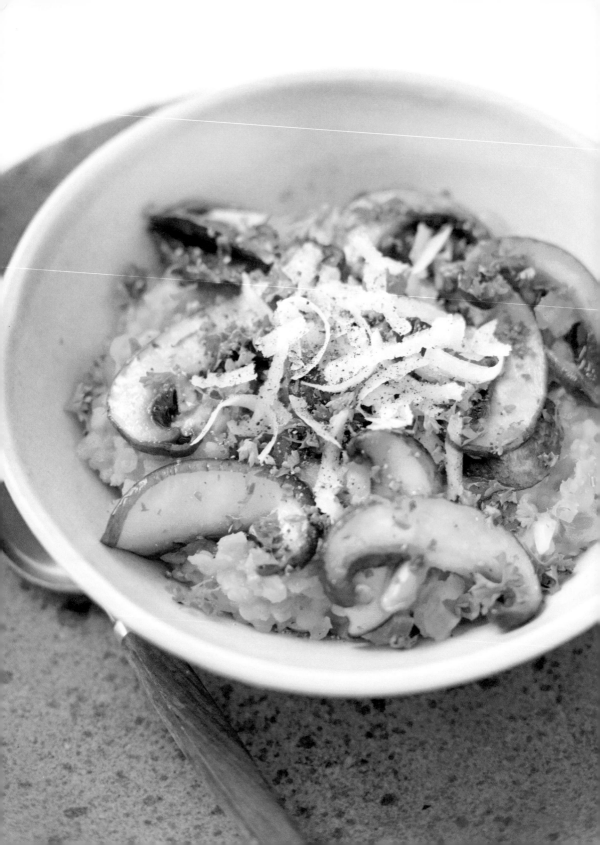

Linsotto with mushroom

One of the nice things about linsotto – which is a risotto of lentils in place of rice – is that the cooking time is short, and it doesn't need stirring the whole time as risotto does. This simple dish tastes great and is a nutritious alternative to the classic risotto dinner. It tastes good on its own or as an accompaniment to meat or fish.

SERVES 1

200 g (7 oz) lentils
2 garlic cloves
½ onion
1 handful of mushrooms
butter or oil, for frying
400 ml (14 fl oz) water
1 teaspoon organic vegetable stock powder (without MSG)
grated parmesan cheese, to taste, plus extra to serve
chopped herbs, to garnish

Rinse the lentils well. Crush the garlic and chop the onion. Cut the mushrooms into slices and set aside.

Add a little butter or oil to a frying pan, followed by the lentils, garlic and onion. Let it all sauté for 3–4 minutes until the onion is soft and glossy. Add the water and stock powder, and cook the lentils until they are tender, around 15 minutes.

Stir the grated parmesan into the lentils.

Add a little butter to a frying pan, and fry the mushrooms for 2 minutes on each side. Stir the mushrooms into the linsotto and serve sprinkled with grated parmesan, some chopped herbs and salt and pepper to taste.

5

6

7

8

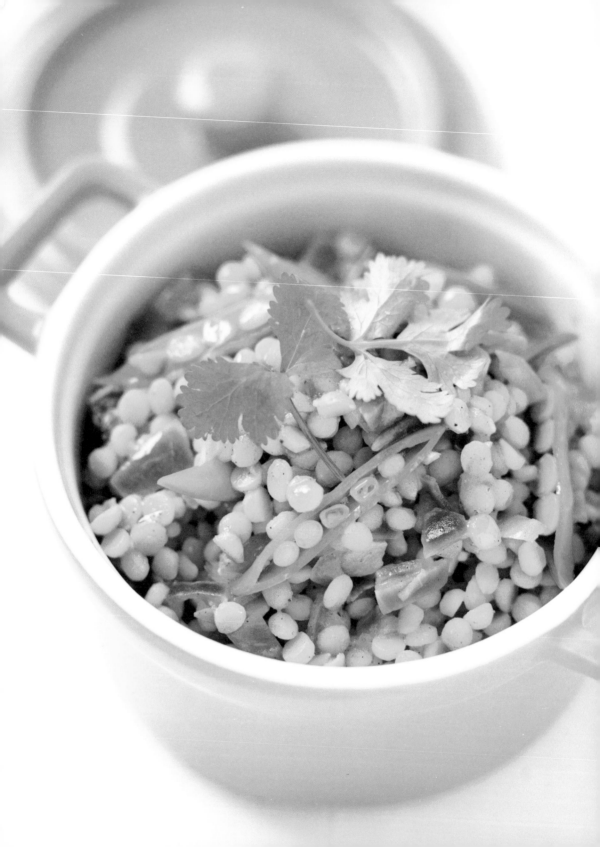

Indian dal

This dish is full of spicy flavours and is a good, filling alternative to rice and potatoes.

SERVES 4

450 g (1 lb) yellow lentils
1 litre (35 fl oz/4 cups) water
2 garlic cloves
1 red onion
1 green chilli
2 tablespoons extra virgin olive oil
1 × 2 cm (¾ inch) piece ginger, finely grated or shredded
1 teaspoon ground cumin
2 teaspoons ground turmeric
2 teaspoons garam masala
1 tablespoon organic vegetable stock powder (without MSG)
100 g (3½ oz) fresh coriander (cilantro) leaves
100 g (3½ oz) snap peas or other greens, such as cabbage, green beans or broccoli
1 teaspoon ground coriander
¼ teaspoon ground cardamom
juice of ½ lime
sea salt and freshly ground black pepper

Put the lentils and water in a pan. Bring to the boil and let the lentils cook for 10 minutes. Chop the garlic, red onion and chilli.
Heat the olive oil in a frying pan, and sauté the garlic, red onion, ginger and chilli for 3–4 minutes until the onion is soft and glossy, being careful not to burn the garlic. Stir in the cumin, turmeric and garam masala and fry for 1–2 minutes until fragrant.
Drain 500 ml (17 fl oz/2 cups) of the lentils' cooking water into a bowl, and stir in the vegetable stock powder.
Pour the stock over the onion mix in the frying pan. Drain the rest of the cooking water from the lentils, and add the lentils to the frying pan.
Chop the coriander leaves, and cut the snap peas into strips. Stir the fresh coriander, snap peas, ground coriander and cardamom into the lentils.
Season with the lime juice, salt and pepper.

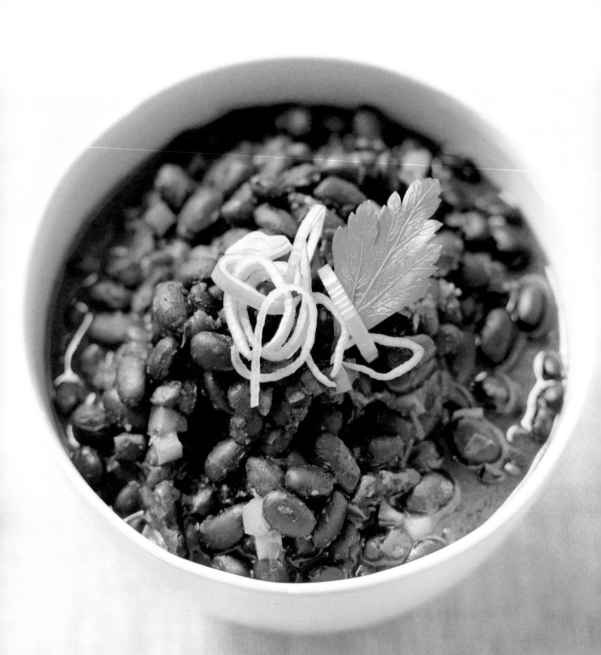

Black beans

This is a very simple twist on the typical black bean stew that is served in Cuba. The flavour is gentle and rounded with a certain sweetness, and goes well with both meat and fish.

SERVES 4

250 g (9 oz) dried black beans
1 green capsicum (pepper)
½ large onion
3 garlic cloves
1 bay leaf (optional)
1 teaspoon dried oregano (optional)
1 teaspoon ground cumin (optional)
sea salt and freshly ground black pepper
balsamic vinegar (optional)

Let the dried black beans soak in about 1 litre (35 fl oz/4 cups) of cold water. Leave them at room temperature for at least 12 hours, preferably longer. I put them to soak the evening before I use them, so it's quick to make dinner the next day.

Drain the soaking water. Fill a saucepan with about 1 litre (35 fl oz/4 cups) of fresh water, add the beans and bring to the boil. There should be about twice as much water as beans, but the amount varies according to how much water the beans have soaked up already. It may be that you need to add a little more water during cooking.

Finely chop the capsicum, onion and garlic.

When the beans are boiling, add the capsicum, onion, garlic, herbs and spices, if using (but don't add the salt yet as it can stop the beans from becoming tender). Turn down the heat so that the stew bubbles away gently. Let it continue to bubble for about 1 hour. After 30–40 minutes, check that there is enough water, and top up if necessary. Cook the beans until they are tender.

Season the bean stew with a little salt and pepper, and the balsamic vinegar (if using). Serve.

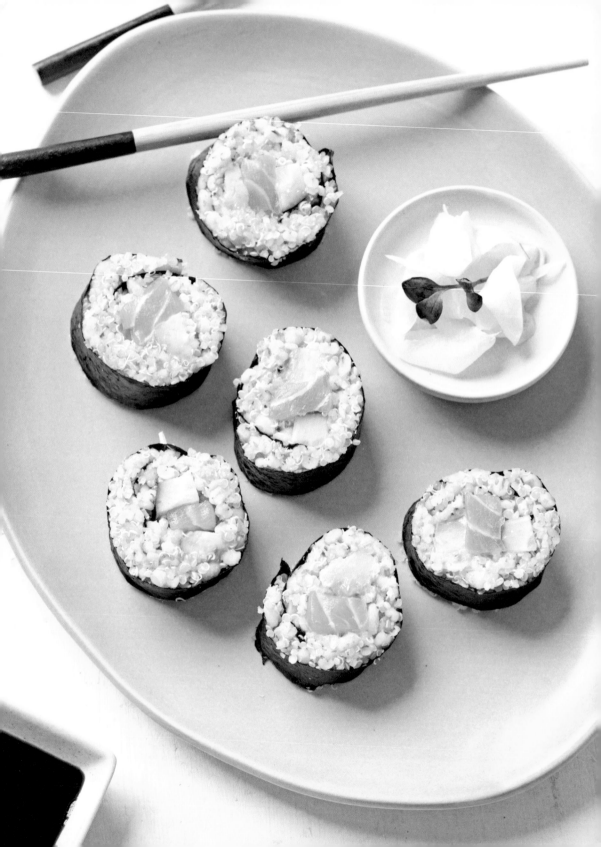

Quinoa makis

MAKES 18–20 MAKI PIECES

150 g (5½ oz) quinoa
3 nori sheets
wasabi
100 g (3½ oz) sushi salmon
1 avocado
⅓ cucumber
fermented soy sauce and pickled ginger, to serve

Note: A bamboo mat makes it easier to roll these.

Cook the quinoa according to the packet instructions. You should get about 600 g (1 lb 5 oz) of cooked quinoa.

Place a sheet of nori at the centre of a bamboo mat, with the short side towards you. You can make makis just as well without a bamboo mat, but it is easier with one. Make sure that the stripes on the nori sheet sit at a right angle to the grooves on the mat.

Spread a tiny strip of wasabi along the top of the nori sheet. Then cover the sheet with cooked quinoa, and press it down well until you have a compact, 3 mm (⅛ inch) thick layer. Don't cover the last 4 cm (1½ inches) of the nori sheet furthest from you with quinoa.

Make a groove in the quinoa parallel to the uncovered nori sheet, 2 cm (¾ inch) from the edge of the sheet nearest to you.

Cut the salmon, avocado and cucumber into 5 mm–1 cm (¼–½ inch) thick strips. Place the strips in a line in the groove.

Use the bamboo mat to roll the nori sheet tightly around the filling.

Leave the roll to rest while you make rolls from the rest of the ingredients.

Cut each roll into 2–3 cm (¾–1¼ inch) thick slices.

Dip the maki pieces in fermented soy sauce, and eat them with a little wasabi and pickled ginger.

5

6

7

8

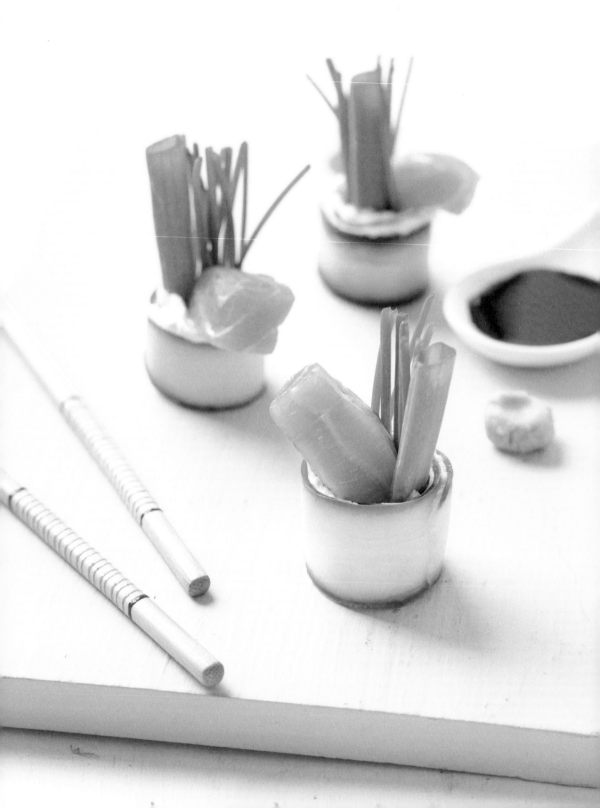

Cucumber makis

MAKES 6 MAKI PIECES

1 small cucumber
3 tablespoons cream cheese
50 g (1¾ oz) sushi salmon
1 small bunch chives
2 spring onions (scallions), the green tips
wasabi and fermented soy sauce, to serve

Shave the cucumber into strips 15–20 cm (6–8 inches) long and 3–4 cm (1¼–1½ inches) wide with a mandolin. Only cut through to the watery core. Turn the cucumber over and shave strips from the opposite side.
Spread the cream cheese along the cucumber strips.
Cut the salmon into strips 1 cm (½ inch) thick and 5 cm (2 inches) long.
Cut the chives and the green tips from the spring onions into 5 cm (2 inch) long pieces.
Place the salmon, spring onions and chives across the cucumber strips about 5 cm (2 inches) from the end of the rolls.
Roll the maki pieces up and place them on a serving dish. In a bowl, stir up a little wasabi with some fermented soy sauce. Dip the pieces in the sauce, and enjoy.

TIP: You can use the rest of the cucumber, spring onions (scallions) and chives in a salad.

5

6

7

8

5 6 7 8

GOAL FOR WEEK 6

In recent years, research has shown that both genetic vulnerability and the bacterial environment in your intestine play a central role in body weight and waist size. This week you are going to learn to include ingredients that strengthen the intestinal flora, so you benefit from fewer health problems, better moods, a clearer mind – and the disappearance of harmful belly fat.

EAT TO ENRICH BACTERIAL FLORA IN THE INTESTINE

As the weeks have gone by you have gradually, almost without noticing it, introduced a daily diet that has not only trimmed your waist, but is also ideal for the microscopic world in your intestine. The billions of bacteria that program your immune system, generate energy and shape good moods are now getting the nutrition that makes them strong. Whereas before they were being weakened by calories from refined foods, they are now transformed with the help of a little honey, fibre-rich grains, vegetables and delicacies from the sea.

Through five weeks of inspiration from effective food tips, both the bacteria and you have received a new boost. Sugar that weakens the bacteria has been replaced with honey, which strengthens them. Refined flour has been swapped for fibre-rich whole grains, which they love. More plant energy is finding its way to your stomach throughout the day, and more fish and seafood is already on the weekly menu.

The helpful bacteria in your intestine also have many more important tasks than just breaking down the food that you eat into smaller units for absorption in the intestine.

Over the last few years, researchers all over the world have discovered the surprising abilities of the intestine's community of bacteria.

I must admit I believed that they were all just loose theories the first time I read about them, and that they had no scientific backup. It wasn't until a colleague of mine took his PhD in the same bacterial communities that I became more convinced. When I think about it again, both my personal experience, and the experience of my patients, is that worries and fears settle in the stomach. Anxious patients all talk about the infamous 'knot in the stomach', and I have personally experienced that stomach bugs and diarrhoea can literally weaken concentration and motivation. Even if we still don't fully understand how it all works, I have come to conclude that we have enormous potential to influence our own health by playing on the same team as our community of bacteria.

In pure figures, the bacteria might make up around 90% of the cells that are found in our bodies. In other words, the intestine is an extremely important organ, which it pays to take care of. The community of bacteria in your intestine communicates with the body and mind. The day-to-day situation in this community affects your immune system, concentration, memory and mood.

The intestine's community of bacteria communicates with the body's cells via hundreds of chemicals. They send messages by using both hormones and neurotransmitters. More than 90% of the body's serotonin – a neurotransmitter that produces happiness – is found in the intestine. It's no surprise that some researchers have begun to call the intestine 'the second brain'.

Countless different bacteria live in your intestine, and you have your own individual, unique bacterial world – so you have your own special profile. Bacterial diversity is called, in technical language, the 'microbiome', which communicates with the brain through long nerve fibres, neuro-transmitters and hormones, and influences the metabolism, the production of insulin, the immune system, the concentration, the mind and the memory (Foster 2013, Kau 2011). If you think the brain governs all, you should probably think again.

How is your own unique microbiome formed, and where do these central players come from? When you first come into this world, you are swarmed by helpful bacteria via your mother's birth canal. Gradually, your intestinal flora are enriched by bacteria that you get from body contact, breastfeeding and the many things you put in your mouth. Babies lick and suck for fun, and toddlers eat sand. When I was little, I loved the taste of carrots straight out of the ground. I only wiped them off in the grass before I sank my teeth into them. They were full of bacteria that, if suited to my microbiome, became a permanent fixture in my intestine and still live there – as long as they get the nutrition they need. Eventually you may have thousands of different kinds of bacteria that perform slightly different functions, and which work together to keep you fit, happy and full of energy.

The bacteria in the intestines need good growing conditions to stay alive, multiply and thrive. They want foods they can ferment (or dissolve) in order to keep themselves alive and become strong – cauliflower, root vegetables, onions, garlic, ginger and oily fish are ideal foods for bacteria.

At the same time, you have to protect the helpful bacteria against unwanted intruders. There are many kinds of unwanted intruders, which easily take control if they are allowed in. These all commonly live off sugar and refined wheat products. If you often choose refined, starch-heavy and nutrient-poor food, the unwanted bacteria can easily take the upper hand. You are simultaneously starving the helpful families of bacteria. The most vulnerable collapse and die out, just as endangered species can perish and disappear entirely from the plant and animal kingdoms. The expertise that they possess also vanishes, so that important tasks are neglected. The immune system gets confused and produces inflammation for no good reason. It may lead to a weakened insulin sensitivity, greater storage of fat, and weight gain. It can also lead to an increased vulnerability to sickness. Furthermore, the brain can get mixed messages and a change in leadership from the intestine. The result can be excess weight, sickness and psychological disorders (Lozupone 2012). Strangely enough, you won't always feel bellyaches, in spite of the warzone in your intestine, but it can have major long-term consequences. An imbalance in the intestine's bacterial community can lead to an imbalance in the mind and body.

WHEN THE BODY IS RAVAGED BY FEVER AND THE IMMUNE SYSTEM IS FIGHTING AGAINST VIRUSES AND BACTERIA, SWEETS AND SOFT DRINKS ARE FUEL TO THE FLAMES. INDULGE IN FOOD FOR YOUR KIND, CARING IMMUNE SYSTEM, AND WIN THE BATTLE SO THE BODY CAN RECOVER QUICKLY!

Danish researchers have investigated the makeup of bacteria in the intestines of 292 Danes in total, of which 169 were overweight and 123 were of normal weight. It demonstrated that people with normal weight had a richer intestinal culture – more helpful, and more varied types of bacteria – than the overweight (Le Chatelier 2013).

French researchers have studied changes in the bacterial makeup of the intestines of 49 overweight people, who were put on a controlled diet. The survey showed that a diet rich in fibre, fruit and vegetables could increase bacterial diversity in the intestine and make it easier to lose weight. So the train has not left the station, yet – you can create changes in your bacterial diversity and enjoy the benefits for your health, weight and quality of life for many years!

Even I learned, painfully, that a relatively short course of antibiotics in autumn could trigger a feeling of sickness in the whole body. I was about to quit the course of pills when I remembered the possibility of taking probiotics. Thanks to beneficial bacteria the nausea disappeared and I started to feel better on the first day, so I was able to continue taking the tablets, while also having enough energy to go to work. I thought, with horror, of how I had lived with such an imbalance in my intestinal flora, and so little energy on a permanent basis, and so I became even more eager to pass on my knowledge of food that enriches the diversity of bacteria and people's lives.

With a weakened bacterial diversity in the intestine, the intestinal lining is in worse condition than usual, and the programming of your immune system weakens. A flood of triggers can stream into the body from such a weakened intestinal barrier. Cells in your immune system are stirred into action for the fight against infection, and they have not learned to quit when the victory is won. Inflammation can spread through your body like wildfire through dry grass. Just as a fire destroys, inflammation damages and destroys tissue. That results in swelling and water retention in the body, weight gain and a weakened sensitivity to neurotransmitters and hormones that make you happy, engaged and focused. Almost all age-related diseases have their roots in inflammation: diabetes, joint and muscle complaints, heart attacks and strokes, dementia and Parkinson's disease.

It's likely that you walk around with an elevated level of inflammatory markers in the blood. Nothing accelerates the ageing process more; destruction caused by the process of inflammation spreads to most organ systems. Several studies suggest that more than 95% of the inflammatory processes in our bodies are due to an insufficient diversity of bacteria in the intestine; the situation down there is much more complex than we once thought.

The intestinal bacteria are partly responsible for the inflammatory reactions in broadly different organ systems. This is expressed as food allergies, asthma, inflammatory disorders in the muscles and joints, autoimmune diseases, type-2 diabetes, cardiovascular disease, mental health problems, weakened concentration, poor memory and/or cancer.

The diversity of your bacteria programs you – when *it* is weak, *you* are weak!

Did you know that your microbiome has gene coding with at least 10 million recipes, while your body's cells can boast barely 30,000? So it's not so strange that your bacterial diversity has a strong influence on your health.

The bacteria in the intestine affect how your body absorbs nutrition, processes chemicals, breaks down starch and fibre, and enhances sensitivity for hormones and neurotransmitters. In short, they affect your day-to-day fitness. Think of it as living in symbiosis with a diversity of bacteria that manage the way you work, even more so than your own genes. They are not just a bunch of lazy so-and-sos. Read on to learn how you can live in harmony with them and create the best conditions for a great life.

Unfavourable bacteria can lead to weight gain

More and more studies make the connection between poor bacterial diversity and weight gain. Different types of intestinal bacteria have different tasks, and they cooperate to program the immune system's cells. A weak diversity of bacteria leads to a fumbled job of the programming that they do, inadequate programming of the immune system's cells and an increased level of inflammatory substances in the body. It is widely known that this weakness leads to a variety of health complaints, but newer studies have further shown that a poor diversity of bacteria causes increased fat storage in the body. By improving your diversity you can lose more kilos of persistent fat.

Bacterial diversity in the intestine is essential for your health, because simple bacteria cannot do the job alone!

Many new studies show that an ailing community of bacteria can even make substances (*lipopolysaccharides*) that create inflammation in your body when they pass into the blood (Cani 2007). They are not just lazy with the programming of your immune system, so that the immune cells create inflammation, but they even create inflammation in the body. That can mean that you walk around feeling that something is not quite right, that you struggle with low energy, suffer from water retention so that your socks leave deep marks in your ankles, and that you lose some of your good mood. So, it's great that you can consume helpful kinds of bacteria to put your community of bacteria back in order. Several research groups are now studying the effect of adding new bacteria to the intestine if its diversity has become a little too barren.

Studies show that the transfer of intestinal bacteria from healthy individuals can improve the effect of insulin in patients with decreased insulin sensitivity and excess stomach girth (Vrieze 2012). That means that the bacteria resume their purpose and that you can benefit from the result. Studies of patients undergoing weight loss surgery have shown that probiotic supplements deliver greater weight reduction (Woodard 2009). You can make it a little easier for yourself to maintain a stable ideal weight by eating foods with beneficial bacterial cultures, and some people will get great help from bacteria in a box, meaning probiotic supplements. They probably won't suit each and every person, but if you can get some benefit from them, they are wonderful.

Foods that can form a rich diversity of bacteria in your intestine are always beneficial; in other words, they can contribute to both a better quality of life and a slimmer waist (Ley 2010).

FOOD FOR A RICH DIVERSITY OF HELPFUL BACTERIA

The complicated thing is that your bacterial diversity is unique to you. The interaction between the microbiome, the immune system and the cells can be disturbed by even the healthiest food. If you are food intolerant, it means that even healthy food like tomatoes, bananas or milk can create waves of inflammation in your body. If you struggle with inflammation-related health problems, you ought to be examined for food intolerance and allergies by a doctor. Also, make sure that you re-establish a rich bacterial diversity in the period after any course of antibiotics, as they can flush out many helpful bacteria for a long time.

RESEARCH HAS SHOWN THAT A DISTURBED INTESTINAL FLORA IN CHILDREN CAN BE RELATED TO EXCESS WEIGHT IN THE FUTURE (KALLIOMÄKI 2008).

Extinguish the fires of inflammation with anti-inflammatory food – for example, green vegetables and food rich in omega-3. Strengthen the maintenance of the intestinal lining with helpful bacteria that it can thrive on. Moreover, avoid foods that trigger intolerance and allergies in you, and choose everyday foods based on pure ingredients with the least possible additives. Choose unsprayed, organic foods whenever possible, to avoid the intake of added chemicals.

Before industrial processing and modern cooling techniques were introduced, we salted, dried and fermented foods for storage. Fish was salted and fermented, as was meat, and berries were preserved in sealed jars. We can brush the dust off earlier generations' fermenting skills, and take advantage of healthy cooking methods – they provide utterly wonderful food. Why not try cured sausage with fermented meat or fish, and kimchi?

In the meantime, there are simpler ways to create bacterial diversity in the intestine. Enjoy porridge or barley oats because these foods contribute soluble fibre, which the helpful bacteria love. Eat more plant greens, all kinds of onions and fibre-rich root vegetables. Oily fish, nuts and seeds, cultured milk and fermented foods with natural bacteria cultures are foods fit for the kings of bacteria.

HIPPOCRATES WAS WELL AHEAD OF HIS TIME WHEN HE DECLARED: ALL SICKNESS STARTS IN THE INTESTINE.

TIPS ON CREATING A BETTER BALANCE
IN THE INTESTINE'S BACTERIAL FLORA

* Eat raw root vegetables – make vegetable spears for evening snacks (see page 149).

* Enjoy oven-roasted root vegetables for dinner – for example, carrots, beetroot (beets) or Jerusalem artichokes.

* Use more cabbage in all its forms: white cabbage, Chinese cabbage (wong bok) or red cabbage. Grate it into salads and add it to raw vegetables, soups and stir-fries.

* Use more fresh herbs: make herb dressings, use flat-leaf (Italian) parsley and basil in salads, add freshly chopped herbs to soups, casseroles and stir-fries when serving.

* Use onions and garlic in many dinner dishes. Make onion salad (see page 151).

* Use more mushrooms in everyday meals. Shiitake mushrooms are a good replacement for chicken fillets. Cook a few button mushrooms with garlic in a frying pan.

* Use more ginger. Make ginger tea for yourself.

* Sneak in a little turmeric in almost all of the dinners you make, such as tacos, chicken curries and stir-fries.

* Use more fresh berries. Frozen berries blended with a little freshly pressed apple juice make a great everyday sorbet that's quick to prepare.

* Select fruit with a low GI, such as apples, pears and plums.

* Treat yourself with cultured dairy products with natural bacteria cultures, like soured milk, Yakult or kefir. Use them in breakfast cereals, smoothies or as a dip.

* Try a probiotic supplement.

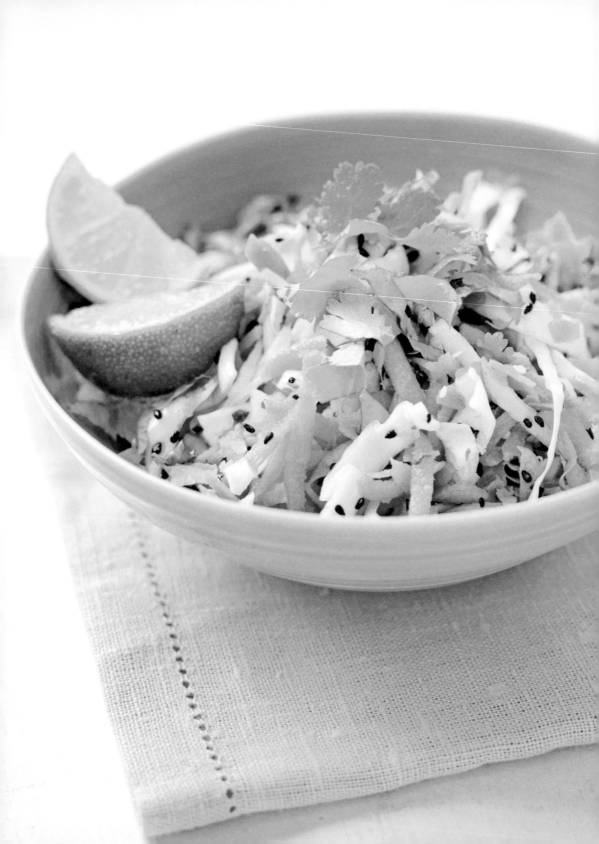

Raw salad with a taste of Asia

Heavenly flavours from Asia turn raw salad into an exciting dish.

SERVES 4

SALAD
3 carrots
1 apple, unpeeled
400 g (14 oz) kohlrabi or turnip
400 g (14 oz) cabbage (preferably a mix of green and red)

DRESSING
4 tablespoons soy sauce
4 tablespoons rice wine vinegar
3–4 tablespoons grated fresh ginger
2 heaped teaspoons forest or heather honey
2 teaspoons sesame seeds – either black or white seeds
about 2 tablespoons finely chopped fresh coriander (cilantro)

Peel the carrots. Grate the carrots, apple and kohlrabi, and shred the cabbage. Put the carrot, apple, cabbage and kohlrabi in a bowl, and mix well. Raw salad tastes really good as it is, without dressing, and is very child-friendly this way.
Mix all the ingredients for the dressing. Pour it over the salad just before serving, and mix together well.

TIP: If you would like to use this wonderful dressing on something else and want a thinner consistency, just add a couple of tablespoons of water to it.

5

6

7

8

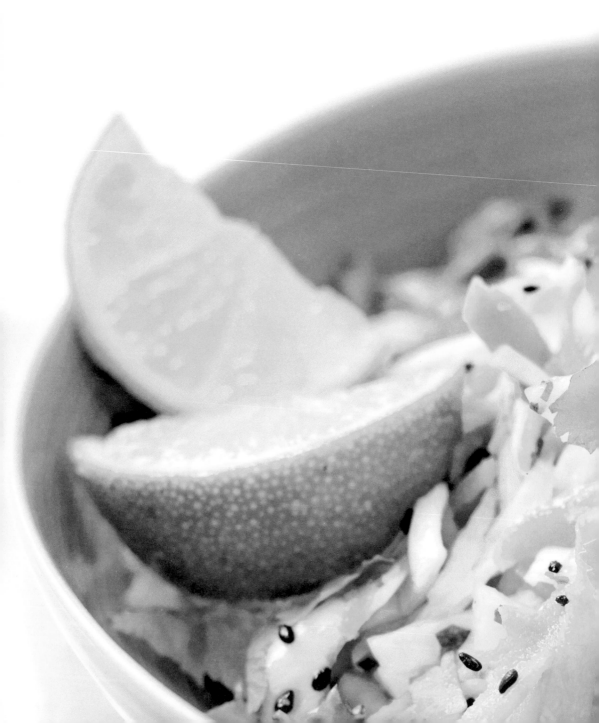

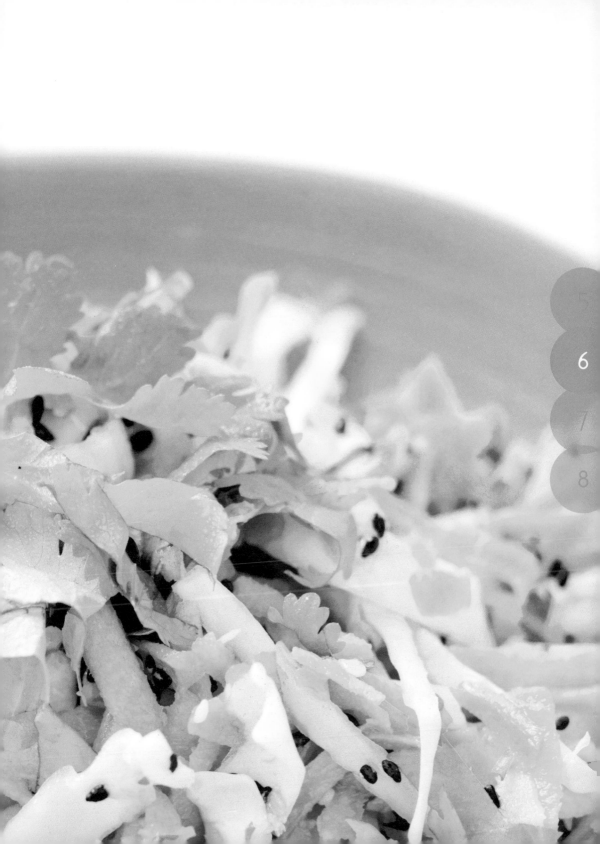

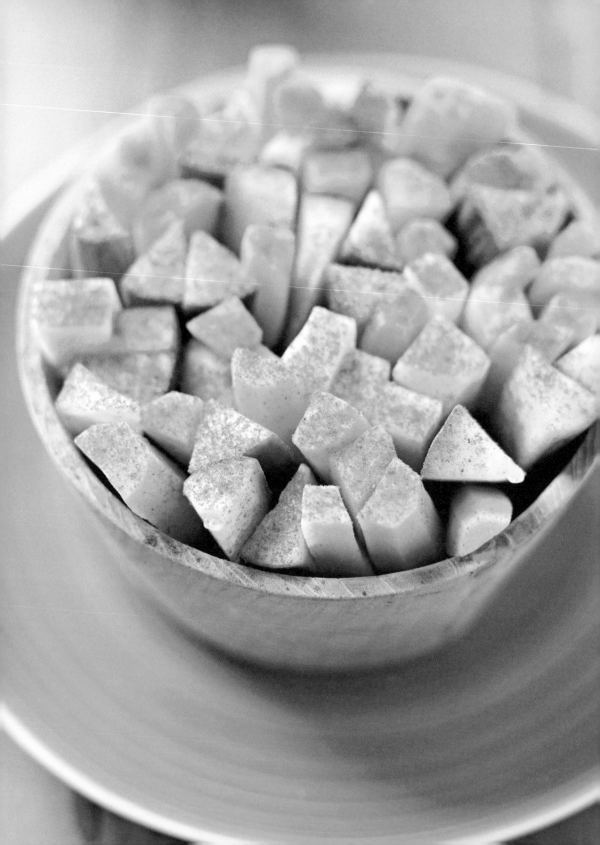

Vegetable spears with chilli

This is a good snack that doesn't need much preparation. Cut up your favourite vegetables and you'll have something good to eat in just a few short minutes.

cucumber
celery
carrot
kohlrabi
cauliflower
zucchini (courgettes)
chilli powder

Cut the vegetables into spears and florets. Sprinkle them with the chilli powder. Arrange the vegetable spears in a glass, and serve with a dip or eat them as they are.

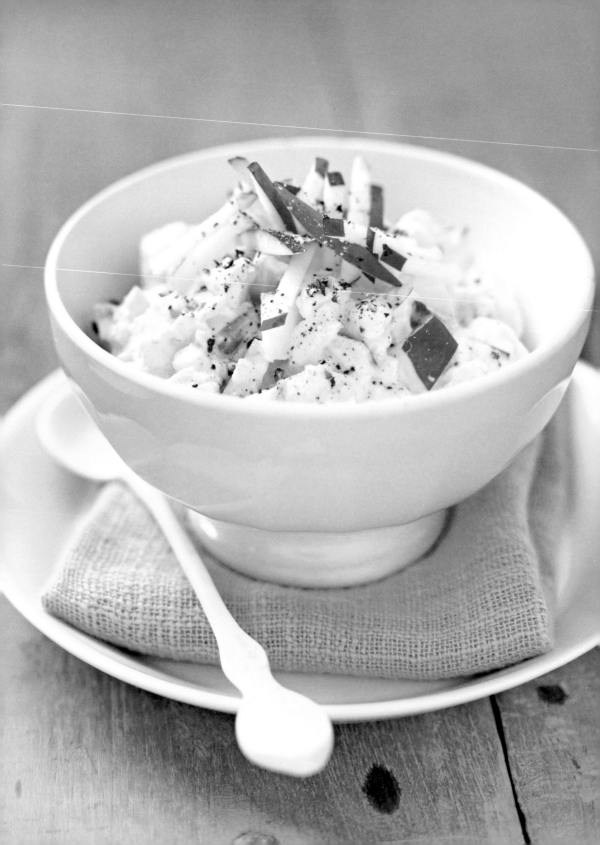

Apple and onion salad

Apple and onion salad is an extremely good accompaniment to both meat and fish.

SERVES 2–3

1 onion
2 apples
100 g (3½ oz) sour cream
curry powder
sea salt and freshly ground black pepper

Chop the onion and apples. Put the onion, apples and sour cream in a bowl, and mix well. Season to taste with curry powder, salt and pepper.

5

6

7

8

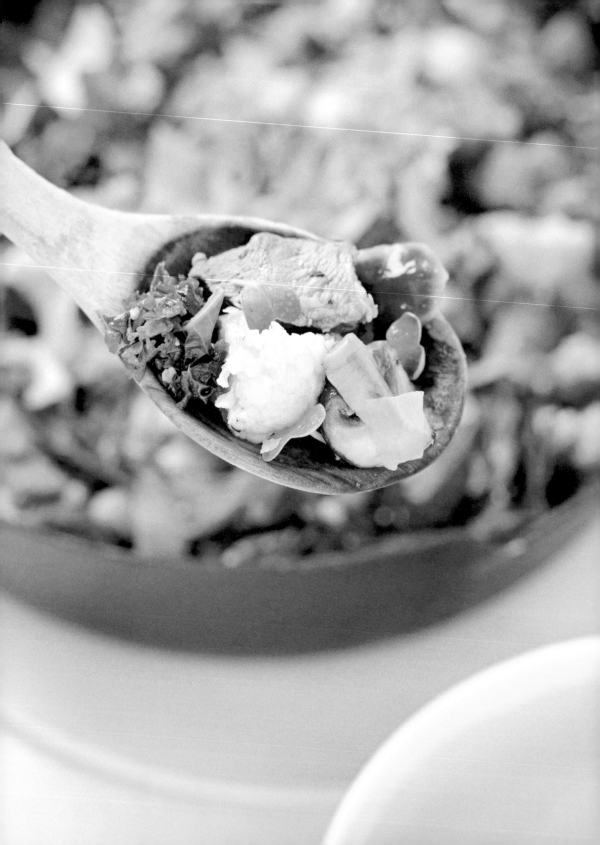

Lamb casserole

This lamb casserole contains lots of cabbage, onion and garlic. It is really tasty, super simple to make, rich in protein, low calorie, child-friendly and cheap. We make it often!

SERVES 6

2 litres (70 fl oz/8 cups) water
2 litres (70 fl oz/8 cups) beef stock or broth, preferably organic beef broth
½ green cabbage
½ red cabbage
1 cauliflower
½ red onion
3–4 garlic cloves
1 tablespoon extra virgin olive oil
400 g (14 oz) diced lamb leg or shoulder (or you can use lean beef or chicken)
10–12 mushrooms, coarsely chopped
pearl barley, wild rice or new potatoes, to serve
thin crackers and butter, to serve

Fill a large saucepan with the water and stock, and bring it to the boil while you cut up the vegetables. Cut the green and red cabbages into strips and the cauliflower into florets. Put the vegetables in the saucepan with the stock. Leave them to cook for 10–15 minutes or until the cabbage leaves are collapsing.

Chop the red onion and crush the garlic. Warm the olive oil in a frying pan over medium heat. Fry the lamb, mushrooms, red onion and garlic for 5 minutes until the meat is browned, then transfer to the saucepan with the vegetables.

Simmer for a further 20 minutes until the meat is cooked.

Serve the lamb casserole on deep plates over cooked pearl barley, wild rice or new potatoes. It also tastes great with thin crackers and butter.

5

6

7

8

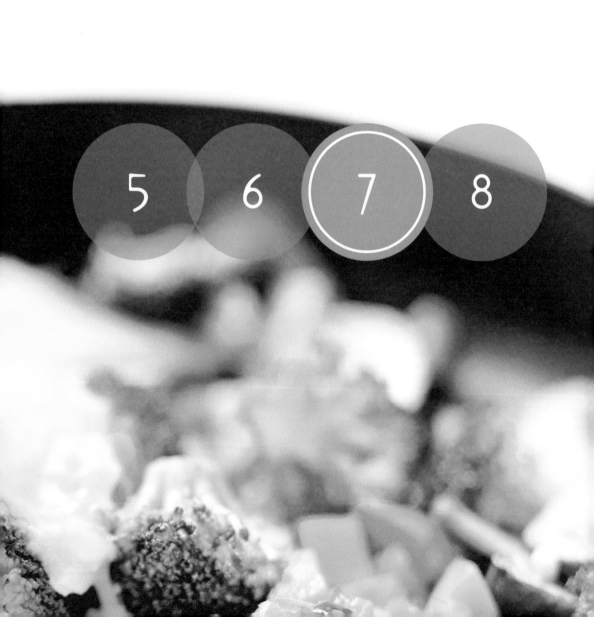

5 6 7 8

GOAL FOR WEEK 7

This week's exercise is to include good sources of protein in all your daily meals. Protein-rich foods provide you with a great feeling of fullness, speed up fat burning and give you stronger bones and muscles. You will be surprised by how a little more protein on your dinner plate lifts your mood and helps you to get rid of belly fat, too.

Eat protein-rich food that provides a feeling of fullness

While last week you focused on giving the helpful bacteria in your intestine the food that makes them resilient, this week you will concentrate on incorporating good sources of protein in all meals. These will be able to give you stronger muscles, a better feeling of fullness and a slimmer waist. Getting enough protein-rich food is important so that you can feel comfortably full, while activating fat burning and losing belly fat. To put it simply, protein-rich meals make it easy for you to lose weight.

Protein provides a better feeling of fullness than carbohydrates and fat – something that cannot be explained on the basis of calorie intake alone. Good sources of protein maintain muscle mass and stimulate fat burning when calorie intake is limited. Protein is, perhaps, the nutrient that increases fat burning more than any other.

And not just that – protein contributes amino acids that turn into the hormones that regulate hunger and fullness. There are good sources of protein in both the plant and animal kingdoms. If you choose protein-rich beans for example, they come with other nutrients that you won't find in meat or fish. If you only choose, for example, soya or meat, it can create an imbalance and a lack of the key contributors to an ideal metabolism. You'll get the best result for your waist measurement and your mental and physical wellbeing by consuming a variety of proteins from plant and animal sources.

In my family of eight, there are three who love meat and don't like the taste of beans. But that's okay. I use a stick blender and whizz the beans into tomato sauces and vegetable purées – out of sight, out of mind.

Proteins are built from amino acids in the same way that words are built from letters. While we have 26 letters in the alphabet, there are 23 different amino acids in food. From these 23 different amino acids, your cells can build connective tissue, muscle fibre and immune compounds, as well as hormones and neurotransmitters that make you feel satisfied, motivated or happy. When you write different words, you use a different number of each letter – you use two p's to write the word 'happy' and two s's when you write the word 'bliss'. When your mood needs lifting in times of stress, for example, more of the tryptophan amino acids are used up relative to other amino acids, so that you can feel comfortable and calm. Different protein sources provide different numbers of amino acids. So, at any given moment, a variety of protein from vegetables, pulses, nuts, dairy products, eggs, meat and fish will best satisfy your need for amino acids.

Amino acid chains join together in the most fantastic, three-dimensional protein structures: beautiful, fluttering braids and wonderful crystals. The cells in your intestinal lining contain the door lock that the three-dimensional structures slide into like keys. When the protein braid unlocks a door, a message is conveyed to the cell. It happens in various ways. Sometimes the lock will open for different chemicals so they can flow into the cell. At other times, the turning of the protein key in the lock triggers chemical reactions in the cell. If the three-dimensional structure is damaged, it is like grinding down the key's teeth – it no longer fits well enough in the lock. Heavy processing under heat and pressure damages the valuable protein structures, a process called denaturing, so that they lose some of their effect – effects that the isolated amino acids can't give. Poached eggs take better care of the protein structures than hard-boiled or fried eggs. In this way, the body is adapted to nature; you get the best results from protein by processing it only gently.

PROTEINS MAKE YOU FEEL COMFORTABLY FULL

When your brain cells make hunger hormones, you get the urge to eat something. You can also feel a craving for food through stress, boredom or the need for comfort. Cravings are not the same as hunger. I get an urge to eat something when I am a bit unmotivated and struggling with an article that needs to be completed, even if I am not hungry. I guess comfort eating is the name for it.

When you have eaten a little, fullness hormones are produced that act as keys in the door locks. You begin to feel full. When this feeling becomes sufficiently strong, you put down the fork. The fullness hormones don't work quite as well in the evening, so it's easier for you to overeat after the sun has gone down. Therefore, eat your evening meal any time before 7pm, or decide to eat until you are a little less full in the evening. It is well known that the eyes are bigger than the stomach – at night, though, it can be the opposite, and the stomach never seems to be fully satisfied.

The composition of your meals, with natural carbohydrates, proteins and fats, is key to keeping the hunger and fullness hormones in good balance. Roughly equal measures of the calories from the various sources on the dinner plate keep unpleasant food and sugar cravings at bay. In this way you will stop having constant urges for one or the other, and will instead feel fully satisfied until the next mealtime comes around.

Did you know that the hunger hormone ghrelin strengthens your sense of smell when you are hungry? That's possibly why we go weak at the knees for the smell of fresh bread, or can't resist the offer of a free bun when we are buying coffee and have the munchies at a café.

Good sources of protein at mealtimes give you a comfortable, long-lasting feeling of fullness and a more stable blood sugar by delaying the passage of the stomach contents down to the intestine. The food somehow lasts longer and is absorbed more slowly, and you get a more stable delivery of nutrients to the bloodstream.

This can completely remove the need for snacking between meals, as well as making you feel more energetic for longer. Maybe you won't feel the need for an afternoon nap any more, but instead will feel the urge to go for a stroll outside.

Maybe you are just one of the many whose batteries run low in the afternoon and evening. You want to go out for a walk, but you can't find the will. Don't despair, because when the calories from refined foods no longer drain you of key nutrients, and seafood and other sources of protein are meeting the cells' needs, your energy levels and mental alertness will soon appear again. I have received many happy stories by email about just that – pure food creates pure energy.

PROTEIN-RICH MEALS SPEED UP FAT BURNING

Several studies have shown that protein-rich diets lead to a greater loss of belly fat and better preservation of muscle mass during weight loss than traditional low-calorie diets (Due 2004). It also appears that good sources of protein can make it easier to stabilise at your ideal weight.

YOU BURN CALORIES WHEN YOU BURN PROTEIN

An increase in the protein content of your diet, even a fairly modest one, can make it easier for you to hold on to a stable ideal weight. A part of the reason is that the body burns energy to break down protein, and you burn calories in the process. More protein and less fats and carbohydrates at mealtimes lead to a higher calorie consumption after eating. This is the so-called *thermic effect* (Halton 2004).

Digesting protein is a big job. Around 25% of the calories in protein are lost to its own digestion, while the digestion of fat and carbohydrates only burn around 5%. Choose protein-rich meals when you want to lose weight.

It's not surprising that an eight-month study of more than 1200 adults, from eight European countries, showed that those who consumed protein-rich diets lost weight more easily and found it easier to keep the weight off (Larsen 2010).

In another study, 100 overweight women were split into two groups that consumed similar amounts of calories for 12 weeks – but one of the groups was fed a more protein-rich diet (34% vs 17% of calories). The protein-rich diet produced higher fat burning so that the women in the protein group lost substantially more fat, even though both groups lost similar amounts of weight (Noakes 2005).

A calorie is not, therefore, *just* a calorie. Consuming higher calories from protein also means that you build up stronger muscles and bones, in addition to losing fat (Westerterp-Platenga 2009).

Let's get to work and include a good source of protein in every meal – breakfast as well as lunch, and any in-between meals. Beautiful snacks like fruit and smoothies can be almost protein-free. I have actually had to use a good dose of imagination to get good sources of protein into snacks and in-between meals. Fruit and berries can be enjoyed together with protein-rich nuts and seeds, or a little cottage cheese. In order to achieve a good balance on your dinner plate, you need two handfuls of plant greens, a handful of starch-rich foods like bread, whole grains, corn or potatoes, and a handful of protein. At breakfast you can sneak in a little more protein with additions like cottage cheese, eggs, fish or protein powder smoothies. Add quinoa, beans, chickpeas, seeds and nuts, slices of egg, fish, meat or diced cheese to salads to increase their protein content.

The balance between hunger and fullness hormones is best kept in check by eating at fixed times. Write down the times of your meals to help you – including breakfast, morning tea, lunch, afternoon tea, dinner and perhaps an evening snack and/or supper. Snacks can be an apple, a carrot, a handful of nuts, a few pieces of dark chocolate, a little yoghurt, a small smoothie or something similar. Keep food away from where you work, so that you have to go to another room to eat. This creates a fixed structure around mealtimes. You can have your coffee, tea or water at your desk. Eat a similar amount at every main meal. Don't save on the calories at breakfast and lunch so you can eat dinner like a king. This way you'll avoid overeating when you're starving because you didn't eat enough breakfast.

Tips for snacks

★ Crackers with salad plus fish or a slice of cheese

★ A small handful of nuts (10–12) or a few pieces of dark chocolate

★ Chunks of honeydew melon and a little cottage cheese

★ 100–150 g (3½–5½ oz) plain yoghurt with apple chunks and crushed seeds

★ A small sliced pear and some pieces of cheese

★ Vegetable spears with dip (sour cream, guacamole, hummus)

★ A slice of ham or turkey and a slice of cheese wrapped in a large lettuce leaf

5

6

7

8

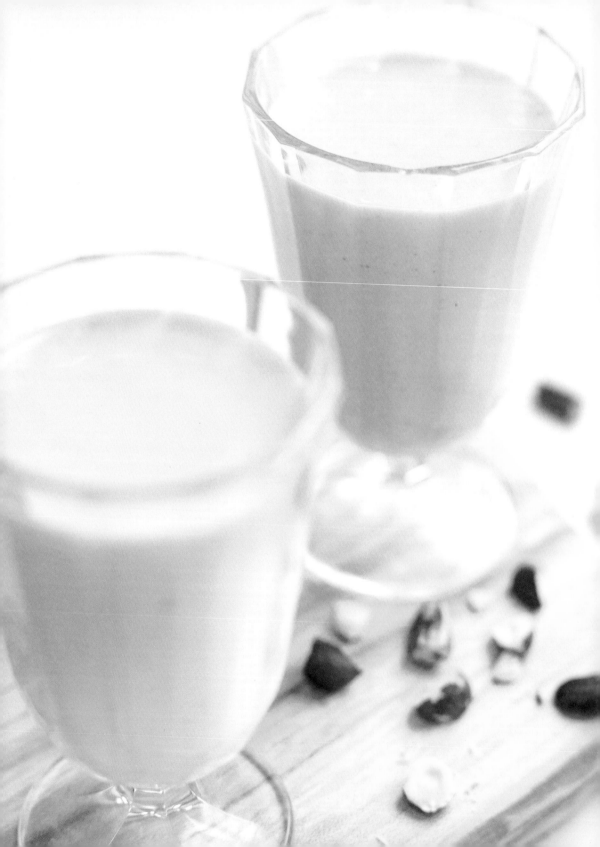

Powderless protein smoothie!

This smoothie has a mild, child-friendly taste with a wonderful sweetness. It's a perfect snack after working out or as a satisfying evening treat.

SERVES 2

100 ml (3½ fl oz) soured milk or buttermilk
200 ml (7 fl oz) organic skim milk
150 g (5½ oz) cottage cheese
1 tablespoon organic peanut butter (or other nut butter)
1 tablespoon freshly ground seed mix
3 teaspoons rolled (porridge) oats
½ banana
1 egg

Mix all the ingredients in a blender at full speed for 1 minute until you reach a smooth, even consistency.

5

6

7

8

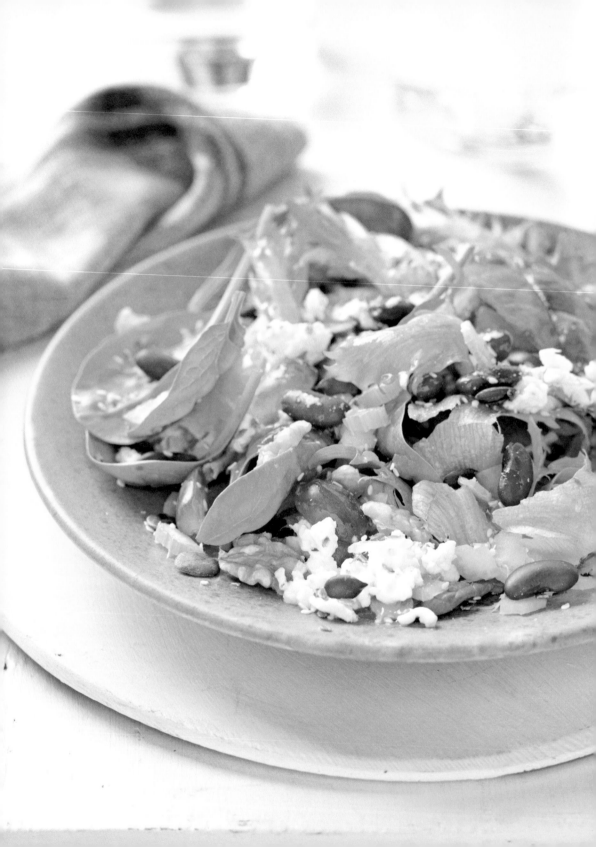

Berit's protein-rich vegetarian salad

Protein from cheese, nuts and seeds make this salad great tasting and satisfying – even without meat!

SERVES 1

2–3 handfuls salad leaves – choose the types you like best
½ celery stalk
8 red grapes
5–6 walnuts
3 tablespoons cottage cheese
100 g (3½ oz) tinned kidney beans or black beans, rinsed
1 tablespoon freshly ground seed mix
extra virgin olive oil and balsamic vinegar (optional)

Tear the salad leaves into smaller pieces.
Finely chop the celery, cut the grapes in half and remove the seeds, if any. Chop the walnuts.
Scatter all the ingredients over the salad leaves.
Drizzle with a little extra virgin olive oil and balsamic vinegar, if you like.

5

6

7

8

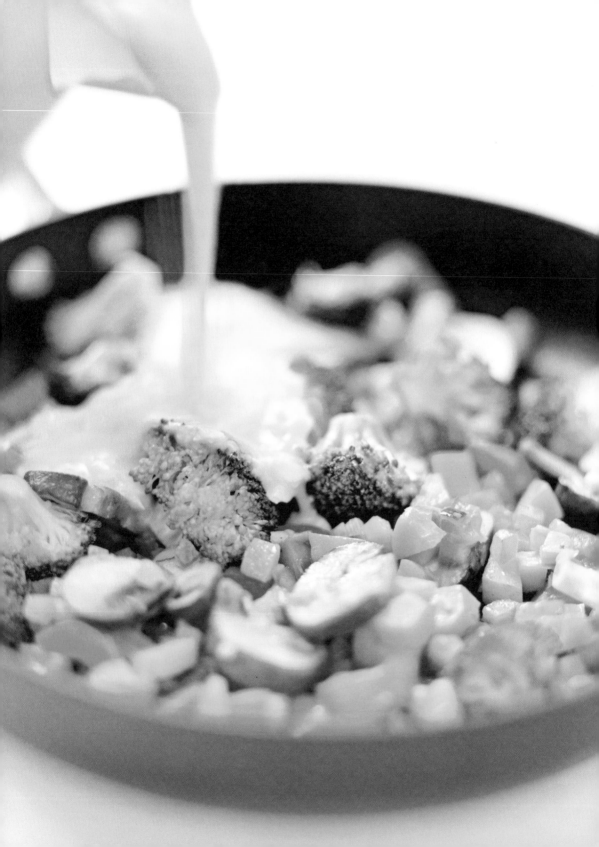

Rainbow omelette

This is quite simply a breakfast full of colours!

SERVES 4

6 eggs
90 ml (3 fl oz) milk
pinch of sea salt and freshly ground black pepper
3–4 mushrooms
½ capsicum (pepper) – you choose the colour
1 carrot
½ red onion
2 garlic cloves
1 small broccoli
2 tablespoons extra virgin olive oil
100 g (3½ oz) grated medium–hard cheese – cheddar or your favourite

Preheat the oven to 200°C (400°F).
Stir together the eggs, milk, salt and pepper in a bowl.
Slice the mushrooms, dice the capsicum and carrot, finely chop the onion and garlic, and cut the broccoli into small florets.
Heat the olive oil in an ovenproof frying pan over medium heat and fry the mushrooms, capsicum, carrot, onion and garlic. Add the broccoli. Let the vegetables soften in the frying pan for a couple of minutes.
Pour the egg mixture into the frying pan, and sprinkle the grated cheese on top. Put the lid on the pan, turn down the heat a little and cook the omelette for 10 minutes. Put the frying pan in the oven for 2–3 minutes to cook a little more on top.

TIP: Use left-over fish, prawns (shrimp) or vegetables in the omelette.

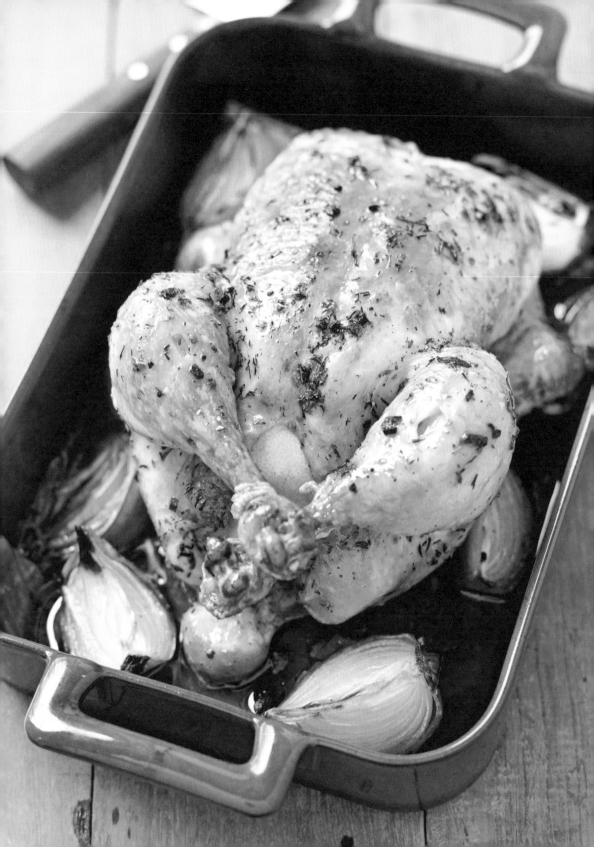

Whole roast chicken

Whole roast chicken is one of the most fantastic Sunday dinners that I know. It's incredible that something so simple and tasty can look so festive! Use organic lemon so that you can avoid pesticides in the zest.

SERVES 4

1 × 900 g (2 lb) organic chicken or turkey
5–7 garlic cloves
2 tablespoons extra virgin olive oil
1 teaspoon dried thyme
½ teaspoon dried rosemary
1 teaspoon sea salt
½ teaspoon freshly ground black pepper
1 organic lemon
2 brown onions
200 ml (7 fl oz) organic chicken or vegetable stock

Take the chicken out of the fridge about 30 minutes before use. You'll get the best result when it's at room temperature. Heat the oven to 225°C (440°F) while you prepare the chicken.
Crush 1–2 of the garlic cloves. Make a herb mix with the crushed garlic, olive oil, thyme, rosemary, salt and pepper. Rub the chicken well with the herb mix.
Prick the lemon with a fork, and cut the remaining garlic cloves in half. Fill the chicken cavity with the lemon and garlic. Sit the chicken in an ovenproof dish. Cut the onion into segments, and put them in the dish. Pour over the stock.
Put the chicken in the oven, and turn the temperature down immediately to 175°C (350°F). Roast the chicken for about 45 minutes. Preferably use a cooking thermometer to check if the chicken is cooked – the meat is ready when the internal temperature reaches 68°C (155°F) and the meat juices run clear.

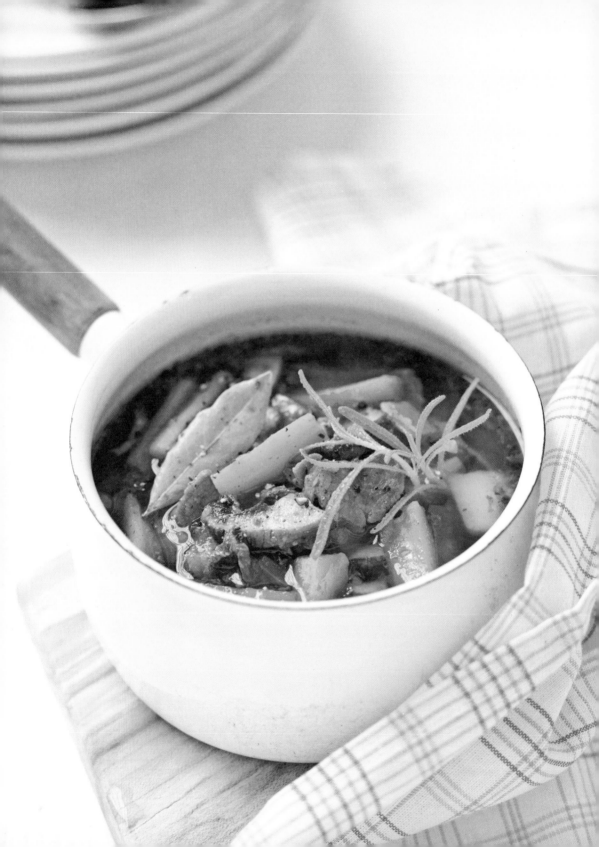

Game casserole

There are many fantastic recipes for game casserole, but this one really scores points because it's so easy to make.

SERVES 4–6

750 ml (26 fl oz/3 cups) beef stock, or
  organic stock cubes dissolved in water
400 g (14 oz) game, for example venison leg
1 large brown onion
4 garlic cloves
2 tablespoons extra virgin olive oil
sea salt
400 g (14 oz) mushrooms
4 carrots, about 400 g (14 oz)
1 turnip, about 100 g (3½ oz)

2 celery stalks
4 tablespoons balsamic vinegar
  or 100 ml (3½ fl oz) red wine
1 teaspoon crushed juniper berries
1 bay leaf
2 teaspoons dried thyme
1 teaspoon dried rosemary
freshly ground black pepper
5–6 small boiled potatoes
cranberry sauce (optional), to serve

In a large saucepan, bring the stock to the boil, and leave it on a low simmer.
Cut the meat into small pieces, and finely chop the onion and garlic. Put the olive oil in a frying pan over medium heat, then fry the meat, onion and garlic with a pinch of sea salt for 5–6 minutes. Transfer the meat and onion mixture to the pan with the stock.
Dice the mushrooms, carrots and turnip, and cut the celery into pieces. Add the vegetables to the casserole.
Stir in the balsamic vinegar, herbs and spices.
Let the casserole simmer until the meat is cooked through and tender (this could take up to 1 hour – start checking after 40 minutes or so).
Take the casserole off the heat. Season with pepper and salt.
Serve with boiled potatoes and cranberry sauce, if you like.

5

6

7

8

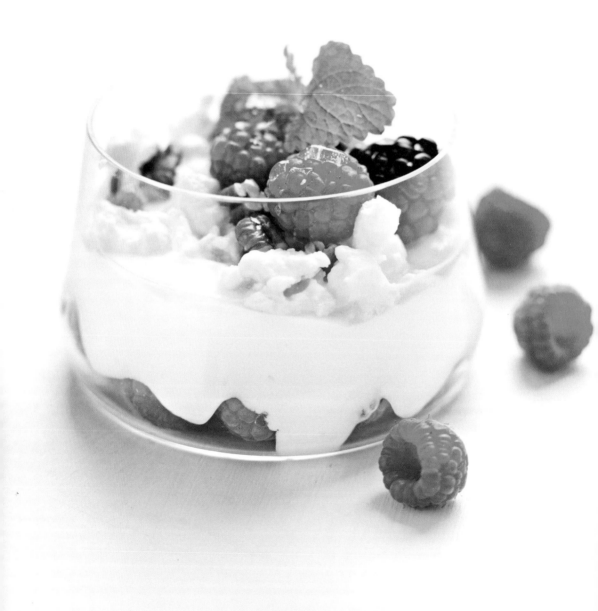

Yoghurt and cottage cheese dessert

This is the simplest dessert in the world: sweet and awesome.

SERVES 1

2–3 tablespoons plain yoghurt
2 tablespoons cottage cheese
about 7–10 fresh or frozen berries
4–5 chopped unsalted nuts, such as pecans or walnuts
1 teaspoon honey
mint (optional), to garnish

Fill a small dessert bowl or a beautiful glass with yoghurt and cottage cheese, and place the berries and nuts on top. Drizzle the honey over the nuts and berries and garnish with mint, if using.

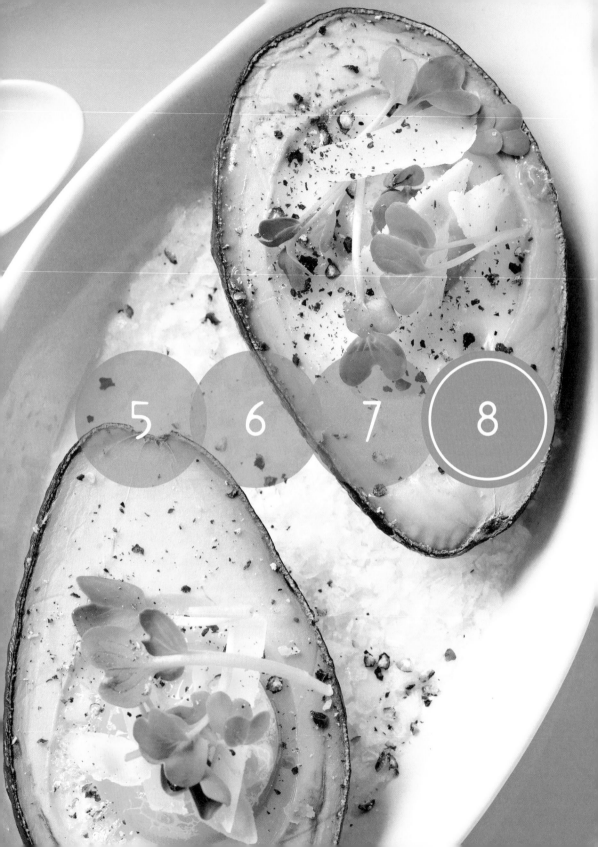

GOAL FOR WEEK 8

This week's exercise is to replace the vegetable oils that increase the amount of harmful belly fat, with oils and foods that are rich in fats that actually cure aches and pains, improve memory, switch on fat burning and give you a slimmer body. There is not just one kind of fat and not all vegetable fat contributes to better health.

USE OIL AND FAT WITH MORE OMEGA-9

Last week you learned about how good sources of protein can improve the feeling of fullness while increasing fat burning. You got tips on how you can easily sneak a little more protein into breakfast, lunch and snacks. This week you will learn more about fat. Many believe they should stay away from fat, and choose fat-free alternatives. But natural fat can actually contribute to a slimmer, fitter body. There is not just *one* kind of fat; it is the kind of fat that matters.

The fats that you see as marbling in a rib eye steak, or as vegetable oil in a bottle, are composed of different kinds of fat. Words like triglycerides (TGL), phospholipids and cholesterol are all descriptions of fats that are found in food. Your body needs all of them – in the right amounts.

Now I am going to tell you a little bit about how fat is constructed, because if you don't understand this it becomes extremely difficult to make the right choices. Most fats are constructed of fatty acids. There are two types of fatty acids: saturated straight fatty acids, and unsaturated bent fatty acids. Mono-unsaturated fatty acids have *one* bend, and polyunsaturated fatty acids have *many* bends. The number of bends in a fatty acid determines what the cells can use them for. Among other reasons, you need saturated fats to maintain regular cell functions, a strong immune system, effective cleansing of the liver, and hormone production. Therefore you should not steer clear of saturated fats, but make sure that you get natural saturated fat in reasonable amounts. Unsaturated fats, like omega-3, omega-6 and omega-9, are liquid at room temperature. When they are built into your cell membranes it becomes easier for the cells to absorb nutrients. Omega fatty acids are used in different ways, from lubricating the walls of the intestine and the blood vessels, to keeping the blood flowing, securing the function of the brain and keeping the memory at the peak of its powers.

Your body needs unsaturated fatty acids of varying kinds in order to function, and it must get omega-3, omega-6 and omega-9 in sensible quantities. Some omega-6 is easily burned as energy, but take too much of this fat and it will be converted into inflammatory substances. Now you understand how important it is to have a balanced intake of the different fatty acids, so your body can maintain good health.

Extra virgin olive oil

Replace refined vegetable oils with extra virgin olive oil. Extra virgin means that the oil comes from the first precious drops that were carefully pressed out of the fresh olives, and therefore it is the most nutrient-rich olive oil. It is incredibly rich in the mono-unsaturated oleic acid omega-9, which reduces the level of inflammatory substances in the blood and has been shown to limit the amount of fat that settles around the waist. In one study, 11 people with a large waist measurement and an impaired sensitivity to insulin were trialled on three different diets. All of the participants consumed the same number of calories, but followed three different diets, one after the other, for 28 days each. The first diet was rich in saturated fat, the second in mono-unsaturated fat and the third in carbohydrates. The diet that was rich in mono-unsaturated fat resulted in increased burning of belly fat, a reduced level of inflammatory substances in the blood and improved insulin sensitivity (Paniagua 2007). Even though more studies are required before a definite conclusion can be drawn on cause and effect, these results are encouraging.

In addition, extra virgin olive oil is rich in plant nutrients called polyphenols. Polyphenols are not just powerful antioxidants – they have much more important duties than simply putting out sparks in the metabolism. Studies on animals have shown that polyphenols increase the burning of body fat as heat (Oi-Kano 2008) – that means that more stored fat is burned as energy. This is the essential oil for your machinery. Take a bottle of good-quality olive oil for a friend the next time you are invited around for dinner. I have learned to appreciate good-quality olive oils, but I only use them in salads or as a pure dip, and not for bread dough or oven roasting. For those purposes you can use cheaper varieties of extra virgin olive oil because the taste is not so important.

Inflammations are usually a good thing. They help the immune defences to keep the pressure up, are a tool in the battle against infections and they clean up damaged tissue. When inflammatory reactions are needed, an army of immune cells is readied for battle or for repair. When the crisis is over, the anti-inflammatory substances quit the fight, so calm can once again take over.

Too many omega-6 fatty acids, however, raise the level of inflammatory substances to unnatural heights, so the body is on guard for no good reason. They can, among other things, lead to inflammation of the joints, asthma, auto-immune disorders, weight gain, weakened sensitivity to insulin and increased storing of fat around the waist. The inflammatory substances can also interfere with the brain cells' receptors. Their sensitivity is impaired so that concentration, alertness, motivation, energy, happiness and memory can be weakened. Vegetable oils that are rich in omega-3 and low in omega-6 are the oils for your waist, but also offer a range of wonderful additional effects in the shape of greater mental and physical strength.

The blood test micro- or high-sensitive-CRP (hs-CRP) is a measure of the amount of inflammatory substances you have in your blood.

Limit the intake of omega-6 to a natural level and aim for a ratio of about 2:1 of omega-3 to omega-6. We can probably even tolerate a little more omega-6 when it comes from natural sources like plants, nuts and seeds, and not from heavily processed fats. You'll do well by cutting out all vegetable oils other than extra virgin olive oil or cold-pressed canola. Ready-made dressings and marinades can create challenges here, due to broken fatty acids, a lot of omega-6 and other additives. It's easier than you think to make your own vinaigrette. That way you can stay away from sunflower oil, corn oil and soya oil, which are very high in omega-6.

Also avoid trans fats and hydrogenated or partially hydrogenated fats. You can easily do this by cutting out margarine, fried food and food products where the vague term 'vegetable fats' is shown on the contents label.

GREAT ADVICE FOR SMART USE OF VEGETABLE OILS

* Use extra virgin olive oil or cold-pressed canola oil.

* Restrict the use of oils from nuts and seeds – it's better to *eat* them to obtain their health benefits.

* Eat chia seeds and crushed linseeds – they are particularly rich in omega-3. Chia seeds contain almost five times more omega-3 than omega-6, and linseeds almost six times more. You have to crush linseeds in order for your body to absorb the linseed oil.

AN INGREDIENT'S OMEGA-3:OMEGA-6 RATIO IS NOT THE ONLY FACTOR THAT DECIDES WHETHER INFLAMMATION IS TRIGGERED IN YOUR BODY OR NOT. YOUR SUSCEPTIBILITY TO INFLAMMATION, THE PROGRAMMING OF YOUR IMMUNE DEFENCES, AND THE COMBINATION OF THE VARIOUS NUTRIENTS IN YOUR FOOD ARE JUST AS IMPORTANT. HOWEVER, STICKING WITH COLD-PRESSED CANOLA AND EXTRA VIRGIN OLIVE OIL AND AVOIDING PROCESSED AND/ OR REFINED OILS AND FATS IS A VERY GOOD START.

5

6

7

8

There is not just one type of fat – not even with saturated fat

When we talk about saturated fat as one type of fat, we group together many different sources of fat that have different effects on the body. Saturated fat from processed meats with many different ingredients, such as sausages and sliced deli meat, don't have the same health benefits as, for example, milk or coconut oil.

The various saturated fatty acids come in many different lengths that give them totally different characteristics in your body. Saturated fat should not, therefore, be talked about as one group. The shorter the fatty acid chains, the easier they are burned in muscles and brain cells as energy. Studies actually show that such fats may improve both memory and concentration. Those are the smart saturated fats you get from milk and coconut oil. The long saturated fatty acids are more difficult to burn as energy and are stored as fat in the body.

COCONUT OIL

Almost 70% of the fat in coconut oil is smart, short- and medium-chained saturated fatty acids. Cold-pressed, preferably organic, coconut fat does, however, have positive health benefits. A Brazilian study examined the effect of taking 30 ml (1 fl oz) of coconut oil per day on 40 women with a waist measurement of more than 88 cm (34½ inches), over 12 weeks, relative to the same amount of soya bean oil. Otherwise, the groups had precisely the same diet, consumed the same number of calories, and were equally active. The groups lost an equal amount of weight, but the women who took coconut oil were the only ones who shrunk their waist measurement. In addition, the coconut oil group achieved a better balance between favourable (HDL) and unfavourable (LDL) cholesterol in the blood (Assunção 2009). Other research has shown that coconut fat can improve the sensitivity of your insulin receptors (Han 2007), produce a higher metabolism for several hours after meals, improve the sensation of fullness and lead to a reduced consumption of food (Clegg 2013, Nagao 2010). More and more new and exciting studies are gradually appearing on the effects of coconut oil. Enjoy limited amounts of coconut fat for the taste, your weight, your mind and your body.

Great tips for the daily use of coconut oil

✳ If you don't have fresh coconut, scatter desiccated (shredded) coconut over breakfast cereals and fruit salads.

✳ Round off the taste in soups, sauces and casseroles with a little coconut milk, in the same way that grandma used to with her famous splash of cream.

✳ Stir a little organic cold-pressed coconut fat into rolled (porridge) oats when serving. It gives a wonderful sweetness with a hint of coconut.

Now that you have cleared up the confusion with oils, and understand that the right fat can actually contribute to positive effects on your health, you can enjoy the taste of those exquisite drops. Spend a bit extra on a high-quality oil, in the knowledge that these drops don't stick to the body but they do sharpen the brain.

5

6

7

8

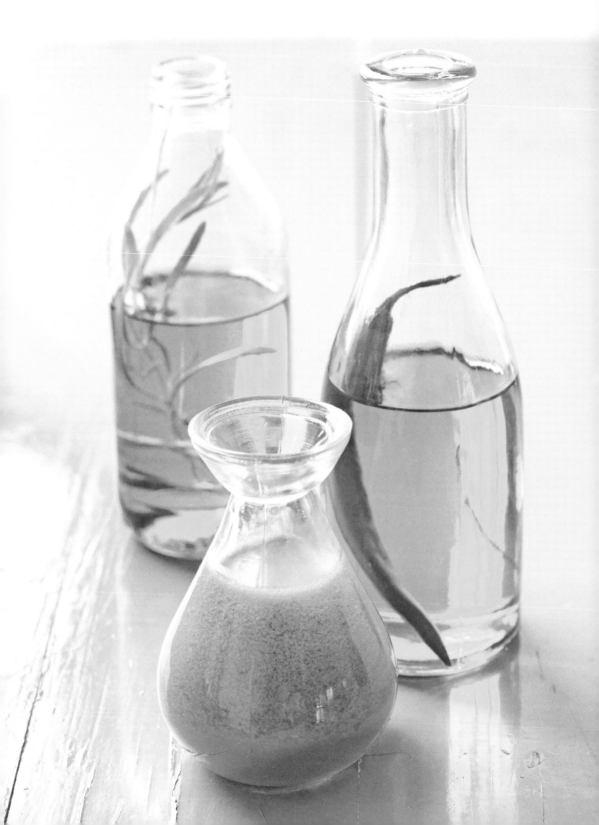

Herb oils

It's easy and fun to make flavoursome oils. Try using herbs and spices that you like. The quality of the oil is crucial to the final result, so choose one that you like the taste of.

AS A STARTING POINT
2–3 herb sprigs, such as rosemary, thyme and oregano, or the peeled zest of 1 lemon,
  1 tablespoon peppercorns, 1 whole fresh chilli or 1 vanilla bean split in half lengthways
extra virgin olive oil or cold-pressed canola oil

Put the herb sprigs, or other flavourings, in a clean bottle, and pour in the oil. Put a cork in it, and put the bottle in a cool place for at least a couple of weeks before you use the oil. Top up with more oil as you use it.

GREEN OIL
100 ml (3½ fl oz) extra virgin olive oil
2 handfuls flat-leaf (Italian) parsley

Put the oil and parsley in a food processor or blender, and blend until the parsley is completely puréed. The oil is super as a flavouring in soups, and also looks beautiful. Drizzle over the soup right before serving.

ROSEMARY OIL
200 ml (7 fl oz) extra virgin olive oil
2 tablespoons dried rosemary
fresh rosemary, to decorate (optional)

Carefully warm up 100 ml (3½ fl oz) of the olive oil with the dried rosemary. The temperature should reach about 60°C (140°F). Let the oil bubble softly for about 5 minutes. Leave it to cool down, and drain it through a fine sieve or similar.

Pour the herb oil into the bowl with the rest of the oil. Mix well, and transfer the oil into a clean bottle. Place a fresh rosemary sprig in the bottle, for decoration.

CHILLI OIL
1–2 fresh chillies
extra virgin olive oil, to cover

Wash and dry the chillies. Cut off the stalks. Put the chillies in a small bottle or jar with a lid, and pour over olive oil until they are covered.

TIP: If you'd like an oil with more kick, you can carefully warm up 100 ml (3½ fl oz) oil in a pan. Then add 20 g (¾ oz) chilli flakes and a couple of whole chillies. Let it bubble softly for around 5 minutes. Leave the oil to cool, then transfer it to a clean bottle or jar with a lid. The recipe can easily be multiplied.

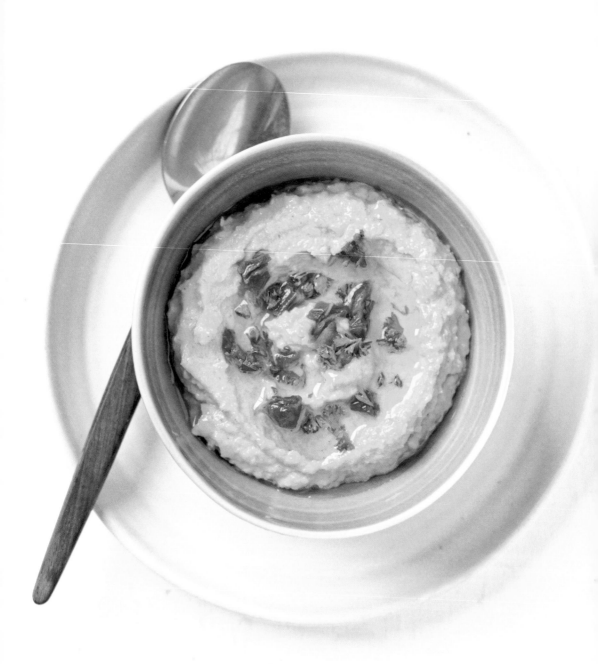

Hummus with sun-dried tomato

You can use this tasty recipe as a dip for vegetables or toasted chunks of bread, on the side with tacos, as a sandwich filling with ham or salmon, or as a sauce for chicken wings in your lunchbox. Protein-rich hummus is a great snack after a training session – a muscle builder at its best.

MAKES ABOUT 225 G (8 OZ)

200 g (7 oz) tinned chickpeas, rinsed and drained
1 tablespoon tahini
1 garlic clove
2 tablespoons extra virgin olive oil
1–2 tablespoons sun-dried tomato
1 teaspoon ground cumin
1 teaspoon ground turmeric
1 teaspoon freshly squeezed lemon juice
1–1½ tablespoons water

Put all the ingredients except the water into a food processor, and blend until everything is thoroughly mixed. Add the water and run the food processor a little more, until you have a smooth, even texture.
Transfer the hummus to a bowl, and serve.

TIP: Try other tasty additions, such as chopped olives, 1 teaspoon paprika, 3 tablespoons organic peanut butter or a little sesame oil. Other variations of eastern spices work well, too – try combining cumin, ground coriander and curry powder. Garnish with chopped flat-leaf parsley and extra chopped sun-dried tomatoes, if you like.

5

6

7

8

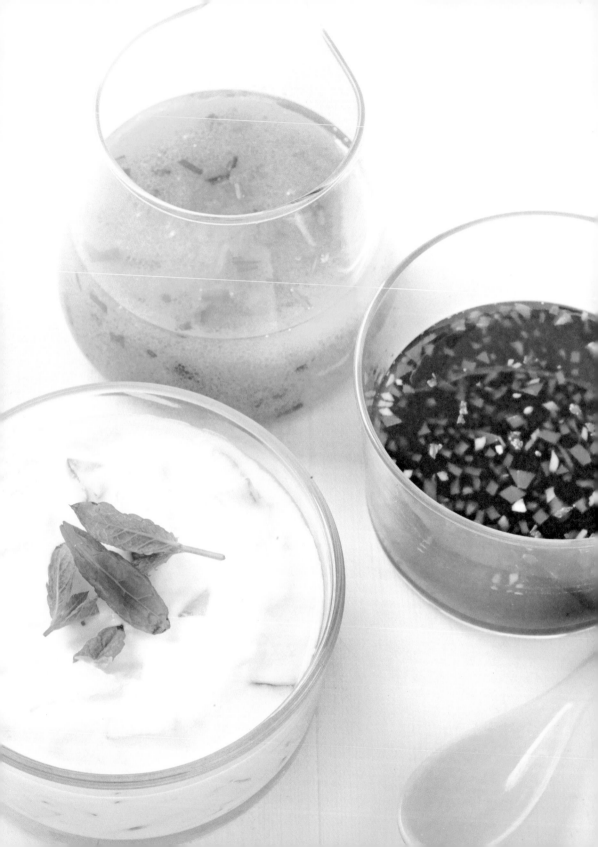

Three great dressings

FRENCH VINAIGRETTE
2½ tablespoons apple cider vinegar
1 teaspoon French mustard
1 teaspoon honey
1 finely chopped garlic clove
pinch of sea salt
100 ml (3½ fl oz) extra virgin olive oil

Mix all the ingredients together, except the oil. Add the olive oil carefully and stir with a fork or small whisk so the dressing becomes thick and luscious.
If you like, add your favourite dried or fresh herbs to the dressing. Try it with finely chopped fresh chives, flat-leaf parsley or basil.

ASIAN DRESSING
2½ tablespoons lemon or lime juice
100 ml (3½ fl oz) soy sauce (preferably with low salt)
½ red chilli, finely chopped
1 × 2 cm (¾ inch) piece ginger, finely chopped
2 garlic cloves, finely chopped
2 tablespoons extra virgin olive oil
freshly ground black pepper

Stir all the ingredients together.

GREEK TZATZIKI
¼ cucumber
150 g (5½ oz) sour cream
juice of ½ lemon
1 garlic clove, finely chopped
sea salt and freshly ground black pepper
mint leaves, to garnish

Grate the cucumber on a large grater. Mix all the ingredients together and season with a little salt and pepper. Garnish with mint.

5

6

7

8

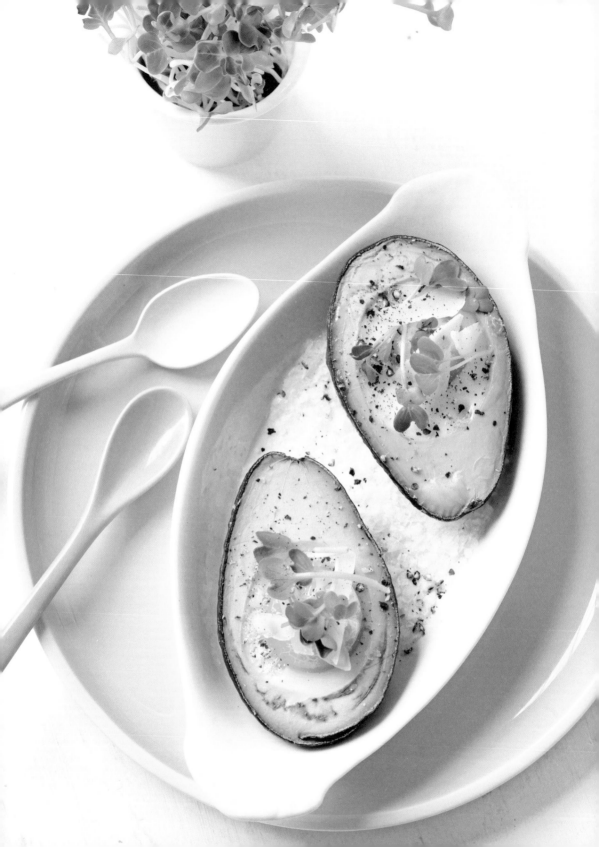

Oven-baked egg avocado

I didn't think it was possible to bake avocado, but just try it – it melts in the mouth!

SERVES 2

1 large, fully ripened avocado
2 organic eggs
1 tablespoon grated parmesan or mozzarella cheese
freshly ground black pepper

Preheat the oven to 175°C (350°F).
Cut the avocado in half, and remove the stone.
Hollow out enough space for the eggs (otherwise they'll run over the side).
Place the avocado halves in an ovenproof dish. Crack an egg into each half.
Sprinkle over the cheese, pepper and your chosen flavourings.
Bake the avocados in the oven for 20–30 minutes until the eggs are set.

TIP: You can use a range of different flavourings with the warm avocado – for example, crispy bacon bits and chives, spring onions (scallions), oregano and chopped tomatoes, thyme, mustard cress and so on. Create your own favourite.

5

6

7

8

WEEKS 9–12

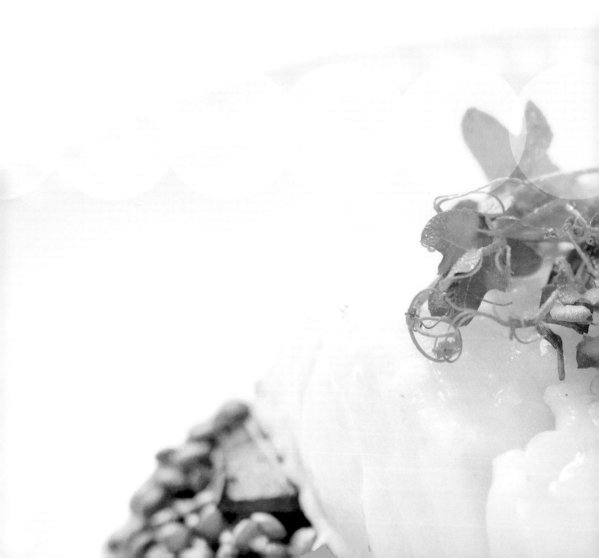

As you start on the last four weeks of this program, you can already revel in the obvious effects on both mind and body. The next four weeks will give you an insight into food and drinks that keep up your great progress. Included are food choices that prevent the return of fat, slow down fat storage and increase fat burning. Fewer health complaints and increased motivation are just added bonuses. Be glad that you have managed to quit calories that *hamper*, and are now eating calories that *pamper*, leading to a better quality of life.

9   10   11   12

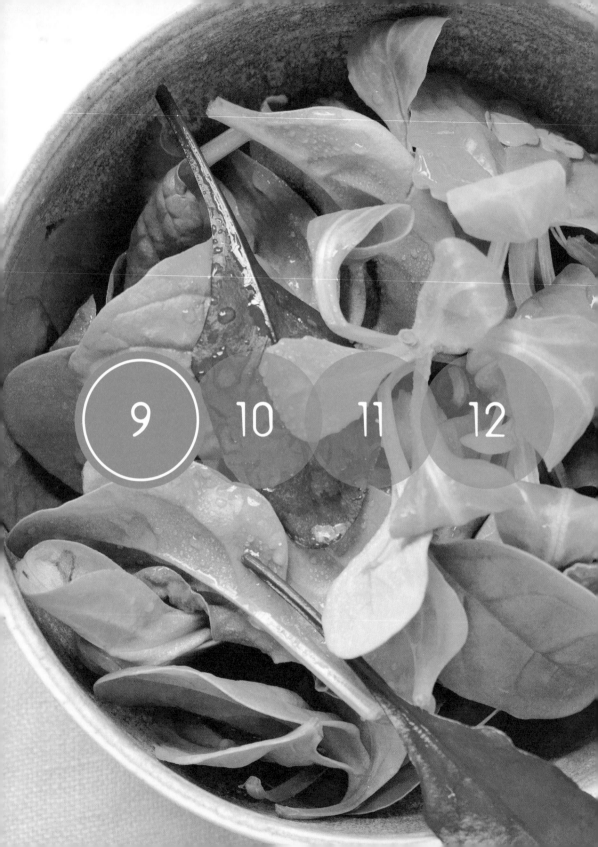

GOAL FOR WEEK 9

This week's exercise is to consume enough of the right minerals. They are your central tools when your cells burn food for energy. This week you are including foods in your daily diet that guarantee you a plentiful supply of minerals. This is so you can build a strong mind and sturdy bones, at the same time as staying on top of your fat burning.

Consume minerals that increase fat burning

The changes that you have carried out over eight weeks are probably the most fundamental in terms of weight and health, but the last four weeks are important too. Even though they concentrate on fine adjustments, you can still underestimate their effects over time. Fine adjustments make it easier for you to eat diversely so that you can secure enough nutrients for yourself, and reach a stable weight and daily diet that you can enjoy for the rest of your life. If you lack minerals in your diet, the effect of these small adjustments is invaluable.

Even though your need for minerals is small, a shortage of them has big consequences. Since they are your cells' central tools, they affect processes in all of your organs.

Without minerals, you can't burn carbohydrate as energy, sustain cell walls, or convert amino acids to immune substances and chemicals for the brain. Essential minerals such as iron, zinc, calcium and magnesium are crucial for healthy functioning of the mind and body. Minerals are chemical elements found in the soil, which is full of them; when you eat plants that have absorbed them from the nutrient-rich earth, they, in turn, enrich you. You can also be indirectly touched by their magic by eating meat, fish, milk, cheese and other products from animals that have eaten the mineral-rich plants.

Poor soil, and the refining of foods, can strip minerals out of the modern diet. When brown rice is made white, wholegrain wheat is converted to white wheat flour, and sugar cane is transformed into white sugar, most of the food's minerals are lost. It has been shown that a range of diseases and disorders in the brain and elsewhere in the body are related to a lack of tools in the cells – increased waist size is no exception.

CALCIUM FOR MORE THAN JUST STRONG BONES

It is common knowledge that calcium is essential for strong teeth and bones, but it is less well known that the mineral can have soothing, slimming and sleep-inducing effects, too. Calcium is essential to life and makes up 12% of your body weight. The mineral controls nerve and muscle function and is used when acids in your body are neutralised. When you know that, you can understand what far-reaching consequences a lack of calcium can have. Nearly all of us have too little of this mineral (Ebeling 2013, Totland 2012) – that's food for thought.

Are you lactose intolerant? Don't despair! There are plenty of great non-dairy sources of calcium, including almonds, walnuts, sesame seeds, pepitas (pumpkin seeds) and green vegetables. However, you would need to eat a lot of nuts and vegetables to cover your 1000 mg daily requirement of calcium, so most people with milk allergies or intolerances probably need help from calcium-enriched food or supplements.

Several studies indicate that the consumption of dairy products such as milk, yoghurt and cottage cheese leads to increased fat burning and the building of stronger muscles. In one study, much greater weight loss (-5 kg) was observed over the course of 12 weeks when three portions of yoghurt were included in a reduced calorie diet, when compared to a reduced calorie diet alone. The yoghurt group achieved a considerably slimmer waist than the other group (-4 cm vs. -0.6 cm). The drop in waist fat was more than 80% greater in the yoghurt group (Zemel 2005). Another study showed that a diet rich in calcium from dairy products can reduce the uptake of fat, and double the flushing out of fat from the intestine (Bendsen 2008).

Different nutrients can probably take the credit for the effects of dairy products. A variety of players deserve a mention: short- and medium-chain saturated fatty acids (see page 179), proteins (see page 156) and different minerals like calcium and magnesium (Van Loan 2009). Branched-chain amino acids (leucine, isoleucine and valine) in protein-rich whey are responsible for the muscle-building effect because they provide amino acids to new muscle fibres, and because they influence the production of the growth hormone (Sanders 2012).

If you are limiting your intake of calories for a period of time, it's a good idea to include some dairy products in your daily diet to protect yourself against muscle loss, to save bone mass and to shrink your waist size

9

10

11

12

(Chen 2012, Josse 2012). However, if you choose dairy products with 'added sugar' you will probably cancel out the result, due to sugar's negative effects (see page 22). It's better to boost the effect with natural solutions like soured milk, yoghurt and cottage cheese.

In a 12-week study, 53 overweight college students were split into two groups, where both were given the same amount of calories (500 kcal less than their estimated need). The first group received a supplement of calcium (600 mg) and vitamin D (125 IU). The two groups lost similar amounts of weight, but the group that received the supplement lost significantly more fat mass, especially belly fat (Zhu 2013).

How can it be that calcium shrinks your waist measurement? It appears that calcium can be both 'the chicken and the egg'. If your body is supplied with too little calcium, your skeleton is raided for the mineral. At the same time, your body produces a hormone to increase the uptake of calcium from the intestine. That same hormone causes you to store fat around the waist. If you are getting enough calcium from food, it saves you from activating the hormone and raiding the stores in your bones quite so often. The calcium can actually reduce the absorption of fat in the intestine while increasing fat burning in your fat cells (Bendsen 2008, Zemel 2005).

An increased intake of vitamin D and calcium appears not just to reduce the amount of belly fat – each and every fat cell appears to shrink, too (Caron-Jobin 2011).

We used to think that a few extra kilos on the body produced stronger bones. The theory has, however, been challenged by studies that indicate that increased belly sizes lead to lower bone density and decreased regeneration of bone tissue. Fat around the waist creates inflammatory substances that seem to raid the skeleton for minerals. A big stomach can therefore suggest brittle bones. Studies show a connection between the amount of belly fat and bone weakness in people as young as 12 years old. In a study of girls aged 12–18 years, it was found that the amount of bone mass was inversely proportional to the amount of belly fat (Russel 2010). The more belly fat you have, the less effective the regeneration of your bone tissue. Bone tissue regeneration may be reduced by 64% in the upper weight groups (Cohen 2013).

So, the increased intake of calcium-rich foods can increase the shedding of fat, can speed up fat burning, reduce the waist measurement and build strong teeth and bones. As if that wasn't enough, foods with a lot of calcium can offer even more. Curbed cravings, fewer mood swings and less tiredness in women with premenstrual syndrome (PMS) (Bertone-Johnson 2005) are all big gains along the road to a slimmer life.

It can be tempting to buy calcium supplements instead of changing food habits. As with many things, though, pure ingredients win out over supplements. Research reveals that dairy products, as part of a reduced calorie diet, provide significantly better results for fat burning and body weight than calcium supplements, when following the same diet (Abargouei 2012). In a study of 100 overweight women that ran for eight weeks, the consumption of milk produced greater loss of belly fat than calcium-enriched soy milk or calcium supplements (Faghih 2011). So, focus on a diet that satisfies your daily requirement for around 1 gram of calcium! I have several patients who aren't able to consume enough calcium through pure ingredients. Children, the sick and the elderly can also find it difficult if they don't have much of an appetite. Ask your doctor if it would be wise to take a calcium supplement for a while, but do this in addition to consuming calcium-rich food, not instead of it.

AMOUNTS OF CALCIUM IN DIFFERENT FOODS (PICK SOME FROM THE TABLE EVERY DAY)

FOOD	PORTION	CALCIUM (MG)	KCAL
Milk	200 ml (7 fl oz)	246	-
Plain yoghurt	200 g (7 oz)	254	-
Hard cheese (e.g. parmesan)	2 tablespoons grated parmesan cheese	138	46
Medium–hard cheese (e.g. Jarlsberg)	1 slice, about 14 g (½ oz)	102	49
Feta cheese	25 g (1 oz)	140	75
Cottage cheese	100 g (3½ oz)	65	78
Sardines (with bones)	4 pieces	242	100
Tofu (raw)	100 g (3½ oz)	130	94
Sesame seeds (with hull)	1 tablespoon	88	52
Tahini (sesame seed paste)	1 tablespoon	64	89
Almond butter	1 tablespoon	43	101
Molasses	1 tablespoon	172	47
Green leaves (steamed)	100 g (3½ oz)	99	14
Cabbage (cooked)	100 g (3½ oz)	45	21
Broccoli	100 g (3½ oz)	47	26

(also check food labels for calcium content)

9

10

11

12

SOME CALCIUM-RICH FOODS ON THE MENU CAN SWITCH ON FAT BURNING AND REDUCE THE UPTAKE OF FAT FROM THE INTESTINE. WHEN YOU CHOOSE PROTEIN-RICH SOURCES OF FOOD, YOU WILL ALSO BUILD MORE MUSCLE MASS – THAT SIX-PACK COULD MAKE A REAPPEARANCE. MANY PEOPLE ONLY REDUCE THEIR CALORIE INTAKE TO LOSE WEIGHT, BUT THE RESULT CAN BE LOSS OF MUSCLES BECAUSE THE MUSCLE FIBRES GET BURNED AS ENERGY – WHEN THERE ARE SLIM PICKINGS, THE BODY LOOKS ELSEWHERE. KEEP YOUR BODY IN HAPPY MODE WITH ENOUGH NUTRIENTS BY CHOOSING SMARTER CALORIES. PROTEIN-RICH DAIRY PRODUCTS CAN PRODUCE WEIGHT LOSS WITHOUT LOSING MUSCLE MASS (CRIBB 2006). THE CHERRY ON TOP IS THAT INCREASED MUSCLE MASS ACTUALLY RESULTS IN INCREASED CALORIE BURNING, EVEN WHEN RESTING, SO THAT IT BECOMES EASIER TO MAINTAIN A STABLE IDEAL WEIGHT OVER TIME. SO HOP TO THE SHOPS!

GREAT TIPS TO GET MORE CALCIUM IN YOUR DIET

✳ Replace ice cream on your fruit salad or desserts with a little plain yoghurt and cottage cheese.

✳ Put two slices of cheese on one slice of bread, instead of having another cheese slice on more bread.

✳ Mix a little cottage cheese in with a smoothie.

✳ Use a little milk in coffee. Buy yourself a simple coffee machine so you can enjoy a cappuccino as a treat. Even if coffee reduces the uptake of calcium from milk, at least you are getting something.

✳ Grate parmesan cheese or another type of hard white cheese over salads, omelettes, soups, casseroles and other dishes.

✳ Swap sugary yoghurts for plain yoghurts or sour milk (which you can flavour yourself by adding fruit, berries or a little honey or vanilla extract).

✳ Scatter nuts (almonds, walnuts) and seeds (unhulled sesame seeds or pepitas/pumpkin seeds) over salads, or finely chop and stir into porridge when serving.

✳ Bake walnuts, unhulled sesame seeds and pepitas (pumpkin seeds) into bread or crackers.

✳ Use sardines (with bones) as a sandwich filler.

✳ Sauté green vegetables, such as cabbage and spinach, in the frying pan in a little butter with garlic. Grate a little parmesan cheese over when serving.

✳ You still haven't had your 1000 mg? Add a supplement!

9

10

11

12

Magnesium

Magnesium is absolutely necessary for a well-functioning hormone regulator in the brain. This regulator measures the body's condition and produces vital hormones according to the body's needs, whether they are sex hormones, stress hormones or other hormones. The gland keeps a keen eye on the body's need for stress relievers and calming neurotransmitters. Just like a thermostat, it adjusts the amount of stress relievers and soothing neurotransmitters according to feedback from many different organ systems. Magnesium deficiency can interfere with this sensitive thermostat, something that gradually leads to the body being alarmed and to producing stress-reducing substances day and night – even if you are sitting completely still. For you that can mean a nagging sense of unrest, palpitations, heightened worries, poor ability to concentrate, inferior sleep at night or distressing anxiety. It can also mean a diminished desire for food.

After several years of poor diet, many of my patients have a magnesium deficiency, and a body unbalanced with respect to stress relief and soothing neurotransmitters. When the lack of magnesium is remedied, I often find that both the complaints of depression and disquiet are improved. There's nothing strange about that when you understand the mineral's central role as a tool through which the brain cells produce substances that furnish you with peace and happiness.

Stress, in fact, produces cravings for sugar and calorie-rich food. In the animal kingdom, stress is a signal to the brain that there is danger ahead, and cravings for calorie bombs are natural to guarantee energy so that the animal can flee and save itself from hungry predators. A faulty stress regulator as a result of a magnesium-poor diet in humans creates the same craving, but since we aren't running a mile to escape from a real danger, our unhealthy food choices have an impact on our waist measurement.

Magnesium deficiency is widespread among people with a modern diet, in which many foods are refined. We humans don't deal with it well. Different genetic dispositions make it so that some acquire health problems through a small deficit of magnesium before others do. A diet rich in meat and poor in vegetables worsens the situation, because that creates a level of acidity in the body that leads to increased loss of magnesium through the urine (Rayssiguier 2010).

A low level of magnesium is associated with a range of health problems, increased stomach girth and metabolic syndrome among them (Barbagallo 2007). Metabolic syndrome means that you have several risk factors for cardiovascular disease at the same time, namely a waist measurement that is too large, decreased insulin sensitivity, unfavourable levels of fat in the blood, and high blood pressure. In studies, daily diets rich in magnesium are shown to reduce the risk of metabolic syndrome by more than 30% (He 2006).

Where do you find such magnesium-rich food, and is it only the magnesium in that food that has an effect? Many different nutrients in magnesium-rich foods, such as fibre-rich whole grains and green vegetables, can protect against weight gain and belly fat. Magnesium gets a helping hand from plant nutrients, vitamins and fatty acids. Together they make each other stronger, so that you get a better effect than if the magnesium comes alone in the form of a supplement.

I used to prefer the taste of bright, crunchy salad leaves like iceberg or cos (romaine) lettuce ahead of the more bitter, dark-green rocket (arugula) or English spinach leaves. That was before I understood that the dark-green colour means more antioxidant power, and plenty of magnesium. Magnesium is used in cells when I feel happiness, motivation and joy. I fill myself up with copious amounts of dark-green leaves now, because I want to make sure that my cells have everything they need so that I can enjoy a few more little moments every single day. Treat yourself to the best there is (meaning: a lot of dark greens).

TIPS FOR A MAGNESIUM-RICH DAILY DIET

* Make soups with cabbage and spinach.

* Choose new potatoes with the skin on.

* Eat white fish once a week.

* Use avocado for dips, in slices, in salads or as a sandwich filling (try oven-baked egg avocado, see page 189).

* Soak and cook pulses (lentils, kidney beans, pinto beans and so on) once a week. Store them in airtight containers in the fridge or freezer. Crush them into tomato sauce for pizza or tacos, or use them whole in salads, stir-fries and casseroles.

* Buy organic peanut butter and use it as a filling in sandwiches.

* Bake wheat bran and wheat germ into bread and crackers.

* Stir wheat germ into porridge and breakfast cereal when serving.

* Choose brown rice over white.

* Choose plain yoghurt over yoghurt with 'added sugar'.

* Drink coffee with milk.

* Feast on nuts and seeds.

9

In animal studies, the effect of magnesium deficiency has been tested alone. Lack of magnesium was shown to produce a remarkable increase of chronic inflammatory substances in the blood, reduced insulin sensitivity and an increase in the sparks in the metabolism – called oxidative stress. Magnesium-rich diets curb this inflammatory chaos in both animals and humans (Rayssiguier 2010). So, while magnesium's role in the sea of nutrients is being researched further, we can enjoy nature's haul of magnesium and achieve calmer minds, an improved ability to concentrate, limited health problems and a smaller waist.

10

MAGNESIUM IS FOUND IN EVERYTHING THAT IS RICH IN CHLOROPHYLL, IN NUTS AND SEEDS, PULSES AND DAIRY PRODUCTS.

11

12

Enough magnesium for a good night's sleep

The cells in a little gland in the brain, called the pineal gland, consume magnesium when they make hormones that influence the daily rhythm, moods and spirits. Sufficient amounts of magnesium are crucial for the brain's chemistry – for concentration, engagement, memory, and for a good night's sleep. If you struggle with sleep problems, the risk of weight gain is increased. Could magnesium deficiency be the common theme at the root of many of your ailments?

Animals that hibernate are a good illustration of magnesium's impact on a good night's sleep. When the outside temperature gets low, the animals' magnesium levels rise significantly, and they fall into a deep sleep, or hibernation. In humans, magnesium can play a role in the development of winter depression and poor nightly sleep. It's fantastic that magnesium-rich daily diets can actually set those problems right. In a study that looked at the magnesium content in the daily diets of a group of 100 people over 51 years old, as many as 58% got too little magnesium through their diets (Nielsen 2010). Researchers saw a link between low magnesium content in the diet, and poor nightly sleep, high BMI and a high level of inflammatory substances in the blood. After receiving a magnesium supplement (320 mg per day) for seven weeks, the participants in the group slept better and the level of inflammatory substances dropped.

We know from a series of studies that an increased level of chronic inflammatory substances in the blood has a connection with weight gain, type-2 diabetes, brittle bones, cardiovascular disease, depression, poor memory and a high risk of cancer. Making sure that you eat a magnesium-rich daily diet translates, therefore, into robust health.

Are you among those who eat a lot of fruit, but few green vegetables, nuts and seeds? That way you can easily consume too much fruit sugar and too little magnesium. Even if fruit is a healthy starting point, such an imbalance in the basic building blocks will actually accelerate fat storage around the waist (Rayssiguier 2006). So, look after yourself with everyday food that is rich in magnesium.

Nuts are one of nature's treasure troves, but many believe that they are too rich in calories for those who want to lose inches from the waist. What many don't know is that in the context of weight, not all calories are equal. Nuts are full of mineral tools that can contribute when the cells burn nutrition as energy, and when they produce the hormones and neurotransmitters that create calm, delight, the feeling of fullness and good sleep. Moreover, they feature fatty acids (omega-3 and omega-9) and proteins that curb cravings for sugar. They are full of fibre, slow down the uptake of carbohydrates from the intestine, and help achieve stable blood sugar and a long-lasting feeling of fullness. Studies show that raw, unsalted nuts in the daily diet can reduce the risk of weight gain (Bes-Rastrollo 2009).

GOOD TIPS FOR GETTING A FEW NUTS EVERY DAY

✳ Treat yourself to a handful of unsalted nuts and seeds every single day. Buy yourself a little box that will hold a day's portion. Also put 2–3 pieces of dark chocolate into the box. Take the box with you everywhere you go. Getting the munchies in a meeting or on the way home from work? Yep, you've got the answer right there in your pocket.

✳ Add nuts to your regular bakes, so you get a tasty loaf with lower GI!

✳ Chop nuts and seeds and stir them into porridge.

✳ Mix nuts into smoothies – they get crushed up and are invisible to those who don't like them.

A group of 20 women ate a portion of almonds every day (350 kcal per day) for two weeks. They didn't gain weight, even though they ate a few more almonds. This was most likely because they had less desire to eat other unhealthy snacks (Hollis 2007). Include a handful of wonderful nuts with smart nutrients in your everyday food. Your desire for food will be affected, so that the body balances its own energy use. Fantastic!

Many articles indicate that the intake of nuts is inversely proportional to BMI. That means that you don't gain weight by including nuts in your daily diet. On the contrary, introducing a few nuts as part of a reduced calorie diet leads to greater weight loss (Mattes 2008).

Last, but not least, nuts deter inflammation and improve sensitivity in your insulin receptors. Fat, fibre, plant nutrients, proteins and minerals in nuts work together and result in fewer health complaints, increased wellbeing, weight loss and a slimmer waist (Cacas-Agustench 2010).

Of the minerals that help along the way to a slimmer waist, foods that are rich in calcium and magnesium have shown themselves to be effective in a range of studies. This week you have got some simple tips on how you can guarantee yourself the effect of this mineral richness. With mineral-rich seeds, nuts, seafood and vegetables on the menu you can achieve great results that improve sleep and mood. If you can tighten your belt one more notch, see it as a nice bonus!

9

10

11

12

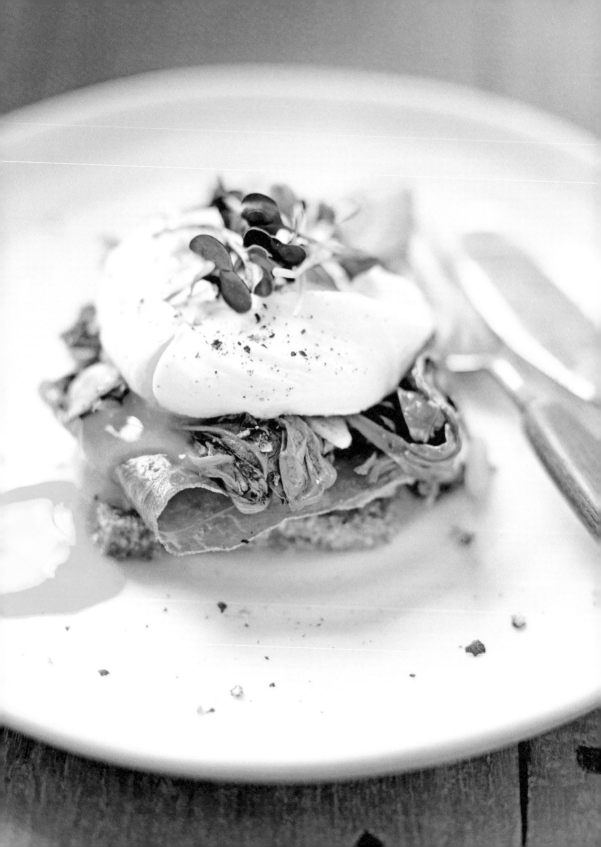

Poached egg on spinach

Both egg and spinach are nutrition bombs with tastes that go well together. The fresher the egg, the better it is. This is one of our breakfast favourites!

SERVES 4

4 slices wholegrain bread
butter
500 g (1 lb 2 oz) English spinach
extra virgin olive oil, for cooking

2 garlic cloves
4 poached eggs (see below)
grated cheese, such as parmesan
sea salt and freshly ground black pepper

Toast the bread and spread a little butter on it while warm. Put a slice of bread on each plate.
Wash the spinach and dry it in a salad spinner or leave it to drain well in a colander.
Warm a little olive oil in a frying pan over medium heat. Chop the garlic, and put the garlic and spinach into the pan. Turn the spinach in the oil so that it collapses.
Divide the spinach among the four slices of toast. Place a poached egg on top, and sprinkle with the grated cheese.
Season with a little salt and pepper.

POACHED EGG
1 litre (35 fl oz/4 cups) water
2 tablespoons vinegar
4 eggs
1 teaspoon sea salt

Bring the water to the boil and add the vinegar. Break each egg into a cup, and season with salt. Keeping the water at boiling point, stir the water round quickly with a whisk so that you get a whirlpool. Remove the whisk.
Quickly bring the cup with the egg over the middle of the whirlpool, and carefully tip the egg in. Hold the water at boiling point for 2 minutes, until the egg white has hardened but the yolk is still soft. Lift up the egg and place it on a sheet of paper towel. Repeat with the rest of the eggs.

TIP: Serve this dish with a few anchovies, smoked salmon, hot smoked mackerel or crispy fried ham, if you like.

9

10

11

12

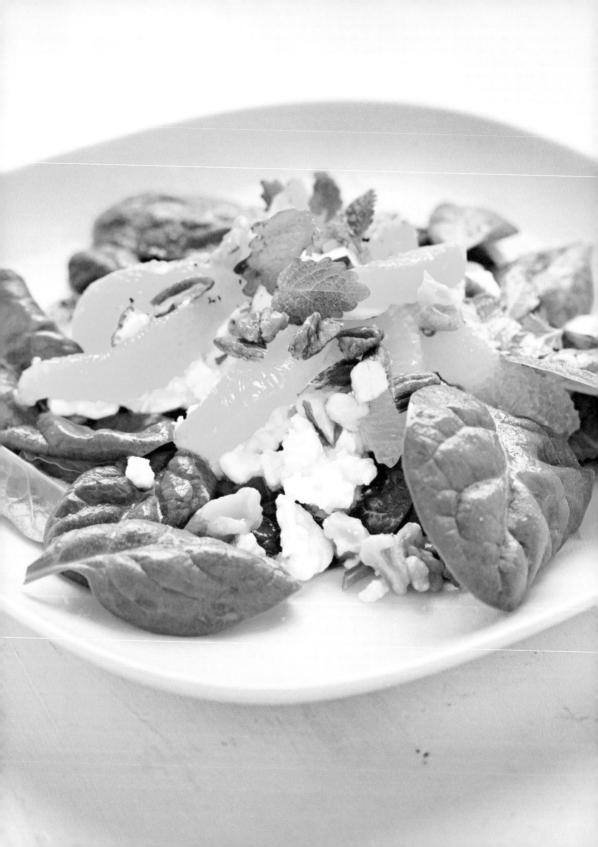

Breakfast salad

Quick, colourful and easy to fall in love with! This delicious salad works for lunch, too.

SERVES 1

2 handfuls mild green leaves, such as baby English spinach or cos (romaine) lettuce
2 heaped tablespoons cottage cheese
½ orange, peeled and segmented
2 tablespoons chopped nuts, such as pecans, almonds, walnuts or hazelnuts
2 tablespoons chopped fresh lemon balm, mint or basil
1 teaspoon honey or maple syrup
sea salt and freshly ground black pepper

Wash, dry and tear the salad leaves, and put them on a plate.
Top with the cottage cheese, orange, nuts and herbs.
Drizzle honey or maple syrup over the top, scatter over some salt, and grind over some pepper.
Serve.

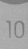

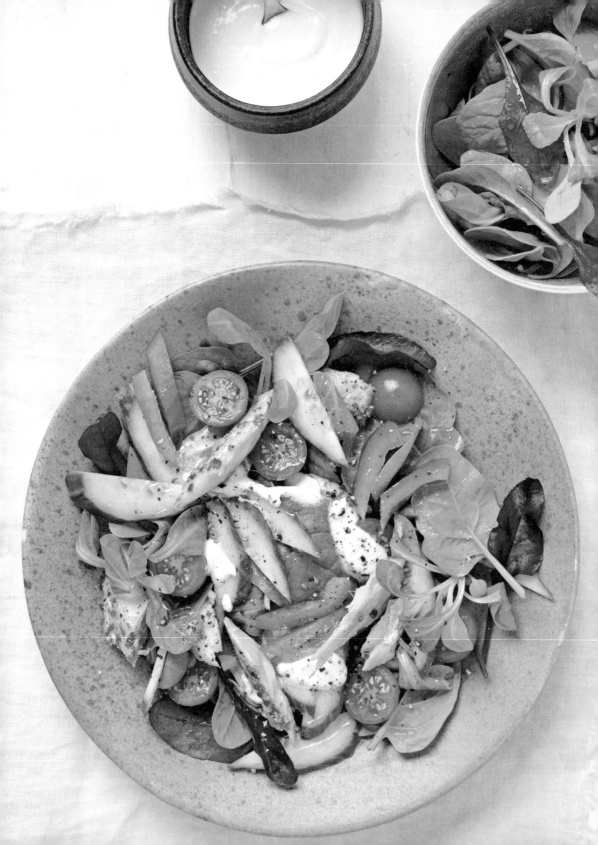

Smoked fish salad

SERVES 2

2 handfuls mixed green salad leaves
½ red capsicum (pepper)
8 cherry tomatoes
⅓ cucumber
2 fillets smoked fish, such as trout or mackerel
sea salt and freshly ground black pepper

DRESSING
3 tablespoons Greek-style yoghurt
squeeze of lemon juice
a little extra virgin olive oil
a little horseradish, to taste
sea salt and freshly ground black pepper

Place the salad leaves on a large dish.
Cut the capsicum into strips, the cherry tomatoes in half, the cucumber into slices and
the smoked fillets into pieces. Combine with the salad leaves.
Mix all the ingredients for the dressing, and drizzle it over the salad.

9

10

11

12

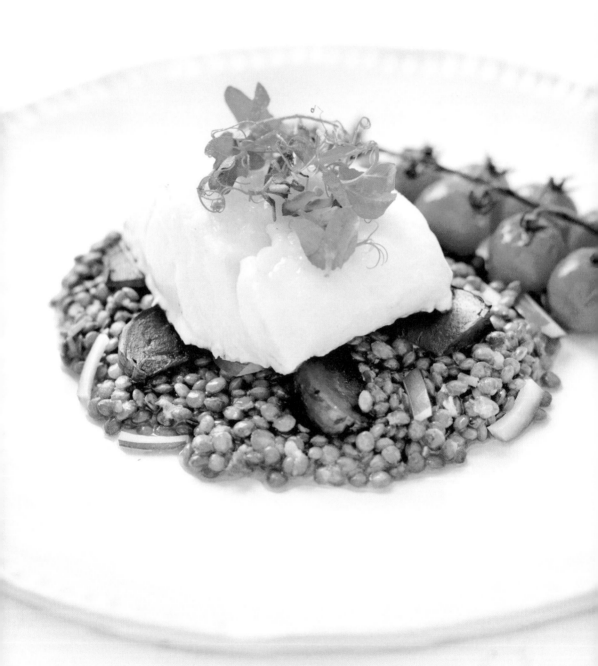

Oven-baked fish with lentils and roasted beetroot

This is a complete fish dinner. Lentil salad harmonises well with the oven-baked beetroot (beets), tomatoes and the fish.

SERVES 4

4 small or 2 large beetroots (beets)
60–80 ml (2–2½ fl oz/¼–⅓ cup) extra virgin olive oil
sea salt
4 firm white-fleshed fish fillets
1 handful small, sweet cherry tomatoes on the vine
300 g (10½ oz) puy lentils or tiny blue-green lentils
2 garlic cloves
1 small red onion
1 small bunch flat-leaf (Italian) parsley
1 teaspoon mustard
freshly ground black pepper
juice of 1 lemon

Preheat the oven to 180°C (350°F).
Wash the beetroots and cut them into wedges. Put them into an ovenproof dish, drizzle over 1 tablespoon extra virgin olive oil and sprinkle a little salt. Bake them in the oven for about 20 minutes, until they are tender.
Meanwhile, place the fish fillets and the cherry tomatoes in a separate ovenproof dish and cook in the oven with the beetroot for 15 minutes.
Meanwhile, cook the lentils according to the packet instructions.
Finely grate the garlic, and finely chop the red onion. Chop the parsley.
Make a dressing of the garlic, mustard and the rest of the olive oil. Season a little with salt, pepper and lemon juice.
Drain the lentils and mix them into the dressing. Mix in the red onion, parsley and roasted beetroot. Serve with the baked fish and the cherry tomatoes.

9

10

11

12

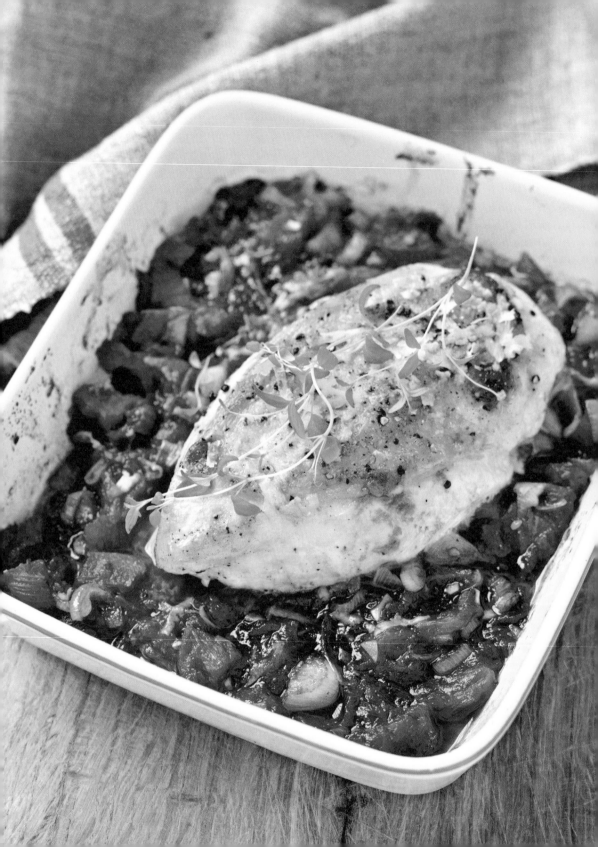

Oven-roasted chicken with tomato sauce

This oven-roasted chicken is easy to prepare in the middle of the week. Tomatoes, balsamic vinegar and parmesan cheese carry the great flavours of Italy. When you choose organic chicken, you are supporting animal welfare at the same time as indulging in the purest possible food, with fantastic flavours.

SERVES 4

4 organic chicken breasts, around 100 g (3½ oz) each
½ onion
2 garlic cloves
extra virgin olive oil, for frying
400 g (14 oz) tinned chopped tomatoes, drained
juice of ½ orange or 100 ml (3½ fl oz) orange juice
3 tablespoons balsamic vinegar
1 teaspoon honey
2–3 teaspoons grated parmesan cheese
1 teaspoon sea salt
freshly ground black pepper

Preheat the oven to 170°C (325°F).
Place the chicken breasts in an ovenproof dish.
Finely chop the onion and garlic. Pour a little olive oil into a frying pan and cook the onion and garlic over medium heat until the onion is soft and glossy, about 2 minutes.
Pour the chopped tomatoes, orange juice, balsamic vinegar and honey into the frying pan, and mix well. Stir the mixture until the honey melts – it happens quickly.
Pour the mixture over the chicken breasts. Scatter the grated parmesan on top. Season with salt and pepper.
Place the chicken in the oven for about 30 minutes, or until it is cooked through.

9

10

11

12

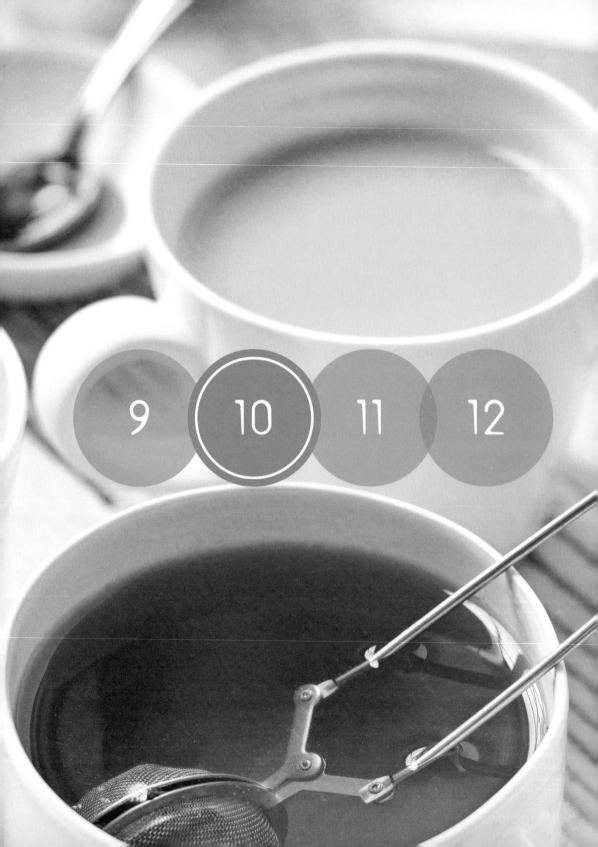

GOAL FOR WEEK 10

This week's exercise is to include green tea and varieties of dark chocolate in your diet. This is because cocoa beans and lightly processed tea leaves provide you with more than lovely flavours – they offer fantastic health benefits, more happiness, energy and a substantially smaller waist.

ENJOY GREEN TEA AND DARK CHOCOLATE

Stabilising your weight, and burning belly fat, isn't just about consuming fewer calories than you burn over the course of a day. It's also about energy and the nutrients that the food can provide. As a doctor, I have had many defeated patients in my office who talk about how little they eat and how the kilos won't budge, no matter what they do. Nutrients in food and drink send signals to billions of cells – messages that control cell divisions and protein production (Jaenisch 2003). The same nutrients can send different signals depending on which other nutrients they are accompanied by. The cells are extremely sensitive to those signals; just see how the body is overburdened when omega-6 damages omega-3, or when your cells are strung out on blood sugar (page 22). Some effects are noticeable the same day, such as changes to your frame of mind. You'll notice the weight after a few weeks, but other effects don't appear for some years, when high blood pressure, diabetes and cardiovascular disease emerge.

If you are putting on the kilos, it can be because you are eating food that is telling your body to turn down the metabolism and store fat. When you make sure that you have a steady supply of the right nutrients, they send sensible signals to your cells so that they increase your metabolism and bolster the feeling of happiness and energy. Good quality of life is the goal – a slimmer waist is just a bonus!

It's not only food that can send these sensible signals. Natural stimulants such as tea and chocolate are also beneficial. When I studied medicine in the 1980s, we learned that the number of fat cells that you have as a one year old will stay with you for the rest of your life. Moreover, we learned that the fat cells are filled with fat and grow when we overeat, and shrink when we starve ourselves. Now, fortunately, we know a good deal more. Your fat cells can obey messages and follow instructions, and they can even decide to die. Cutting calories, on its own, can therefore send completely crazy signals to your fat cells. They may interpret the change as a lack of food, turning down energy consumption and storing fat for emergencies. Don't starve yourself: indulge yourself with foods that give bloated fat cells the hormonal cold shoulder. If you do a little strength training at the same time, you can choose to transform them into muscle tissue and get rid of them once and for all (Zuk 2002). By themselves, low-calorie diets shrink the fat cells because they lose the fat that is burned, but they hold on tight and don't disappear. As soon as calorie consumption increases, they bulk up again. So choose foods that make it possible to transform belly fat to muscle, remodelling the body and leaving you in better health.

Both stress and a lack of nutrients make fat cells swell up. Make space for a few more moments of pleasure in your hectic days. Unwind with treats that put out the sparks and curb inflammation, so your cells can be receptive to the nutrients' magic while transforming belly fat into energy and happiness.

Green tea

Green tea is packed with polyphenols – inflammation-curbing plant nutrients and powerful spark extinguishers. Among them, 'catechins' are well known, but that doesn't mean they can take all credit for the effect. A combination of compounds, including substances we have not yet identified, may be behind the positive effects on health. Studies have shown that catechin-rich green tea increases fat burning (Yang 2012). One example is a study of 60 overweight Thai people, of whom half were given green tea over 12 weeks. The tea group dropped a whole 3.3 kg (7 lb 4 oz) more in those 12 weeks, and their energy consumption increased by an average of 45 kcal/day (Auvichayapat 2008).

It's no bad thing that green tea can also curb oxidative stress, lower the amount of fat that sticks easily to the blood vessel walls, and prevent cancer, diabetes and cardiovascular disease (Wu 2003, Wolfram 2006). Green tea may reduce the uptake of sugar from the intestine and increase insulin sensitivity and the absorption of glucose in the cells. Drinking green tea is a fantastic way to contribute to stable blood sugar, whether you have diabetes or not (Tsuneki 2004).

Even if we only know parts of the story so far, we know a little about how green tea can make it easier for you to maintain a stable ideal weight. It can help you to reduce the intake of food, slow down the absorption of fat and increase the number of calories that are used when you metabolise food (Thielecke 2009). The tea also helps some fat to pass through the body undigested, so it won't feature on your calorie count (Cooper 2005).

While others are studying the merits of tea, you can visit specialist businesses that sell tea and coffee and buy a selection of green teas that you like. Let the people with the experience tempt you with a variety of flavours and learn how you can easily prepare the tea so that you enjoy every single cup. I always carry a few good tea bags with me in my handbag, so I can enjoy an extra good cup of tea wherever there is boiling water – on the train, plane or at work. It leads to so many wonderful moments of pleasure.

Also treat yourself to a big cup of green tea at mealtimes. Drink a little tea both before and as you eat. When you lift up the cup and sip a little hot tea, you are getting short breaks throughout the meal, and feel a growing sense of fullness, so you don't overeat as easily. While a classic aperitif is meant to awaken the appetite, tea helps to slow down the intake of food.

Green tea is the least processed type of tea that you can find, with the most surviving plant nutrients. A whole 30% of the dry weight of tea is polyphenols with strong antioxidant power. Preserve the plant nutrients and the positive health effects of green tea by infusing the tea leaves in water that is not too hot – 70°C (150°F). The benefit is two-fold – this way, the tea doesn't become too bitter, either.

FIVE SERVING TIPS FOR GREEN TEA

1   Infuse green tea with thin slices of ginger and lemon. Add a teaspoon of honey to each cup, stir and serve warm.

2   Make green tea with double the amount of tea. Let it cool, then add a little freshly pressed apple juice, carbonated mineral water and ice cubes.

3   Infuse green tea with fresh herbs such as mint or lemon balm.

4   Prepare green tea with a little honey, and let it cool. Make iced tea with frozen berries rather than ice cubes.

5   Green chai tea: Bring water to the boil and let it simmer for about 10 minutes with a few spices – for example ginger, cinnamon sticks, cardamom, cloves, star anise, vanilla or nutmeg. Then use the spiced water (drained, if you like) to prepare your green tea. Enjoy the tea with a little honey.

Most of the studies of green tea are based on the traditional Asian habit of three cups per day. The tea is just as effective at hydrating the body as water, so you are simply looking after yourself.

Dark chocolate

Dark chocolate also contributes a wealth of polyphenols and many kinds of catechins. A research team was alerted to the cocoa bean's positive health benefits in the 1990s, while they were studying the cocoa-drinking Kuna native people. Drinking cocoa may be a part of the explanation for their exceptionally low incidences of high blood pressure, atherosclerosis, diabetes and cardiovascular disease (Ferri 2003, Hollenberg 1997).

Both cocoa powder and dark chocolate are fantastic sources of polyphenols. These plant nutrients can, among other things, bind themselves to beads of fat in your blood, thus protecting the fat against oxidant attacks so that they don't settle so easily in the blood vessel walls. Consuming cocoa powder or dark chocolate can reduce the amount of oxidants in your body for 2–6 hours (Wang 2000). So trust the researchers' findings and eat a little dark chocolate every day to attain an increased level of spark-extinguishing polyphenols in the blood (Engler 2004). Do not miss out on these fantastically powerful antioxidants that can both slow down the production of irritating inflammatory substances and provide a more effective spark extinguisher. Just imagine that those lovely chocolate flavours can help each one of your cells to keep you a little bit fitter (Mao 2000)!

Treat yourself to dark chocolate and cocoa to get more plant nutrients, which relax your blood vessel walls, so that the blood pressure is lowered. Choose dark chocolate with at least 80% cocoa solids in order to strengthen the defences against the settling of fat in the blood vessels (Wan 2001). The effects of milk chocolate or white chocolate are as good as useless, while dark chocolate pieces can protect you against cardiovascular disease and diabetes, improve insulin sensitivity, smooth out spikes in blood sugar, and soften the surges of insulin (Grassi 2005). Are you one of the many who now feel guilty for not liking its bitter taste?

9

10

11

12

GOOD ADVICE TO SOFTEN THE BITTER TASTE OF DARK CHOCOLATE

* You have to get used to the taste. When you eat a little piece every day, you'll begin to like the bitter taste, because the experience of the taste changes. I had to get accustomed to coffee when I worked on night duty, and it took me two weeks of daily tastings before I liked the taste of both coffee and dark chocolate. Now I can't do without them.

* Don't eat anything sweet before you eat dark chocolate, because then the bitter taste will be even more pronounced.

* Chop walnuts and chocolate and eat them together.

* Melt the chocolate over a water bath together with a little organic, cold-pressed coconut oil. Add some vanilla seeds and a little coconut or grated orange peel. Spread the mixture over baking paper and put the chocolate in a cool place to set.

Animal studies have shown that cocoa can increase your calorie consumption, so that you use a few more calories without any more movement. That means increased weight loss, and it's all thanks to a simple pleasure! Inside your fat cells there are gene codes or 'recipes' that, if they are read out, lead to increased fat storage. Cocoa reduces the readout of those fat-storing recipes, so that you store less fat around the waist (Matsui 2005). That's a fantastic cure wrapped up in a wonderful flavour!

GOOD ADVICE FOR SMART CHOCOLATE PLEASURES IN DAILY LIFE

* Eating around 20–30 g (¾–1 oz) per day is a sensible amount.

* A cocoa content of over 80% contains a good concentration of plant nutrients and less sugar.

* It is better to choose organic chocolate in order to avoid pesticides.

* Look for chocolate with a short list of ingredients.

* Make cocoa drinks with raw cocoa powder, a little honey, water and some milk. Just use a little milk because it slows down the uptake of plant nutrients.

* Make chocolate mousse for parties, desserts or for everyday enjoyment (recipe on beritnordstrand.no).

* Make chocolate nuts to make your daily snacks a bit more interesting (recipe on beritnordstrand.no).

I hope that you have now tried out a few different varieties of green tea, and also have found space for some pieces of dark chocolate. It's better to make rituals of these pleasures, so that you don't forget to enjoy their effects during your busy days. Treat yourself with a cup of tea while you make dinner, and make a habit of breaking off a few chunks of chocolate with your coffee.

These are habits that will help with the suppression of inflammation, that send signals to reduce the storage of fat, lift the mood and boost wellbeing. Let green tea and dark chocolate arouse your tastebuds and conjure up their magic in the mind and body!

9

10

11

12

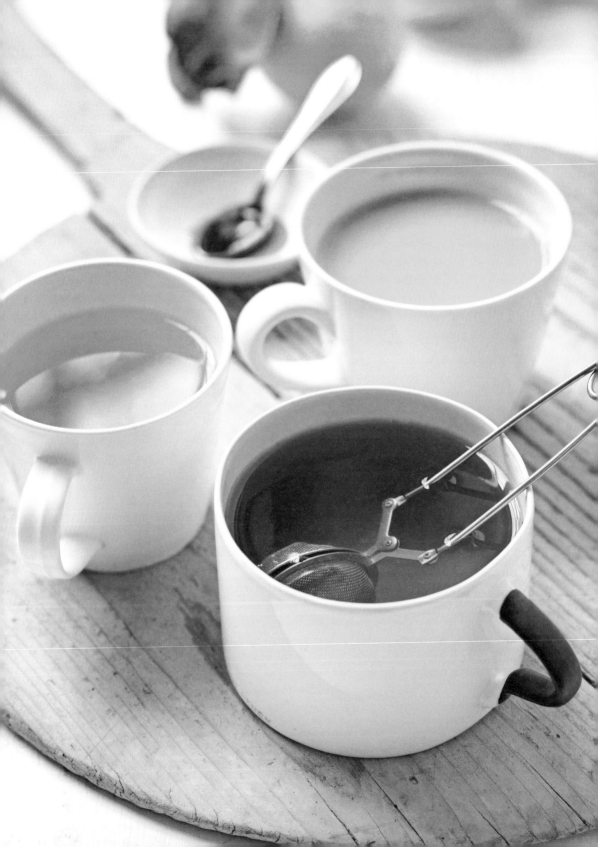

Green tea

Green tea is the best for antioxidant power. Tea comes in many varying qualities. In general, the more you pay, the better the taste and quality. Whether you make tea from loose tea leaves or high quality tea bags, it's likely that you'll get more antioxidants in every sip than if you use cheap tea.

Green chai

MAKES 1 LITRE (35 FL OZ/4 CUPS)

1 litre (35 fl oz/4 cups) water
4–5 ginger slices
1 cinnamon stick
1 star anise
½ vanilla bean, cut in two (don't scrape out the seeds)
5–6 cloves
green tea, in bag or loose
honey, to taste

Bring the water to the boil, and add the ginger slices, cinnamon stick, star anise, vanilla bean pieces and cloves.
Leave it to simmer for 10–15 minutes.
Infuse the green tea in the spiced water (drain the spices if you wish).
Serve the tea with a little honey.

TIP: Add a little steamed cow's, soy, rice or almond milk, if you like. Make enough spiced water for a couple of days – it keeps well in the fridge. Reheat it and let the tea infuse when you feel like another cup.

9

10

11

12

Iced green tea
with mint and lime

This iced green tea sparkles like soft drink, but delivers health in every drop. Use organic tea to avoid pesticides.

SERVES 1

300 ml (10½ fl oz) green tea
½ teaspoon honey
3 lime wedges
4–5 ice cubes
1–2 mint sprigs

Let the tea infuse for 10 minutes.
Stir together the honey and the juice of 2 lime wedges in a small bowl.
Fill a glass with ice cubes and stir in the honey and lime mixture.
Add a sprig or two of mint to the glass together with the last wedge of lime.
Pour in the tea, and stir well.

Green tea with honey and ginger

MAKES TEA FOR 2

700 ml (24 fl oz) boiling water
slices of fresh ginger
2 teaspoons green tea leaves or 2 tea bags
2 teaspoons honey

Pour the water for the tea into two large cups.
Put a few slices of ginger in each cup.
Put the loose tea into two tea infusers or use tea bags. Let the tea infuse for 3 minutes.
Stir in the honey just before serving.

TIP: If you prefer, make green tea with a little squeeze of lime juice, a sprig of fresh mint or lemon balm, a drop of vanilla extract or some berry or fruit juice (not from concentrate) – raspberry and blueberry juice is really good. Don't put milk in the tea because milk proteins seem to interfere with the uptake of healing plant nutrients (polyphenols).

9

10

11

12

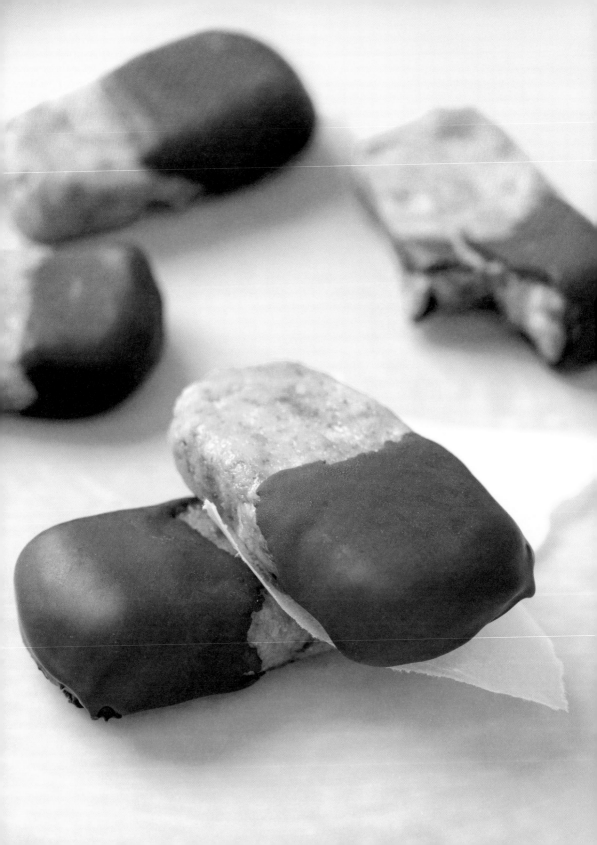

Chocolate and quinoa protein bars

When you get a craving for sugar or just have to have chocolate, this chocolate and quinoa bar is an excellent snack. Quinoa is a fantastic source of protein, giving you all of the nine essential amino acids that the body needs. It's also gluten free and rich in fibre, iron, magnesium, calcium and plant nutrients like quercetin. This is superfood at its best.

MAKES 20 BARS

200 g (7 oz/1 cup) quinoa
10–15 dates or 200 g (7 oz) raisins
200 g (7 oz) raw nuts or seeds, such as almonds, peanuts, hazelnuts, cashew nuts
  or pepitas (pumpkin seeds)
100 g (3½ oz) dark chocolate (preferably 80% cocoa solids)
1 tablespoon organic, cold-pressed coconut oil

Cook the quinoa in boiling water for 15 minutes, pour off the cooking water and leave it to cool. Remove the stones from the dates and discard. Chop the dates in a food processor or blender at full speed for 30 seconds, then set them aside in a bowl.
Put the nuts in the food processor and grind them into nut flour at full speed for 30 seconds. Add the quinoa and dates to the nut flour and process until you get a nice, smooth mixture. Shape the mixture into 20 large protein bars and lay them on a tray. Set them in the fridge or freezer for 1 hour.
Melt the chocolate and coconut oil together in a heatproof bowl placed over a saucepan of simmering water. Dip all or half of each protein bar into the chocolate. Place back in the fridge to harden.

9

10

11

12

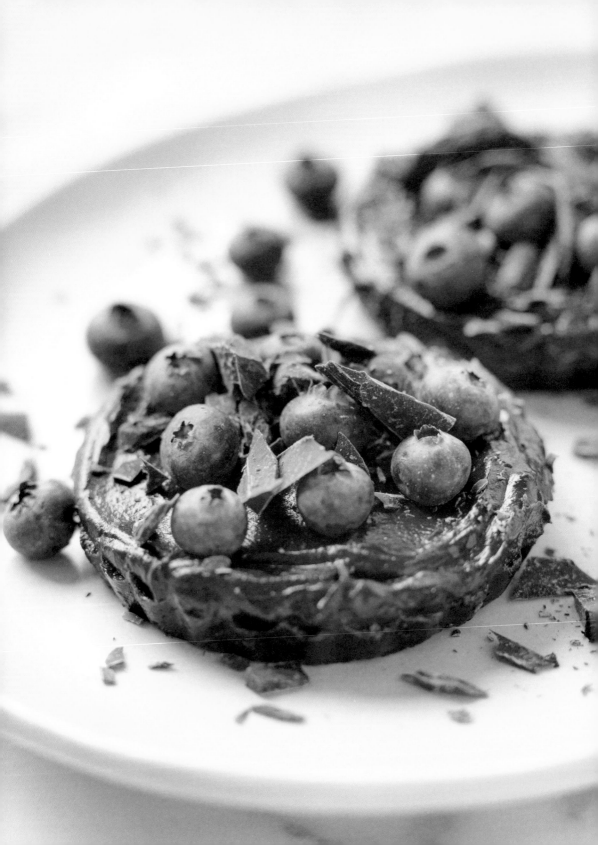

Raw chocolate cake

This is, quite simply, a completely raw dessert favourite packed with nutrients.

MAKES 4–5 SMALL CAKES OR 1 LARGE 20 CM (8 INCH) CAKE

CAKE BASE
500 g (1 lb 2 oz) walnuts
350 g (12 oz) dates, stones removed
1 avocado
pinch of sea salt
1 teaspoon grated organic orange zest
  (optional)
2 teaspoons vanilla extract
100 g (3½ oz) cocoa powder,
  preferably raw and organic

CHOCOLATE CREAM
3 avocados
pinch of sea salt
100 g (3½ oz) cocoa powder,
  preferably raw and organic
100 ml (3½ fl oz) maple syrup

GARNISH (OPTIONAL)
fresh berries
dark chocolate pieces

Finely chop the walnuts and dates. Cut the avocado in half, and discard the skin and the stone. Put all the ingredients for the cake base in a food processor with powerful blades, or use a powerful stick blender and a mixing bowl, and blend together. I mix the ingredients in two or three batches so that the stick blender doesn't overheat.

Line the base of 4–5 individual moulds or ramekins with baking paper and divide the cake mix equally between them.

For the chocolate cream, cut the avocados in half and discard the skin and stones. Blend the avocados, sea salt, cocoa powder and maple syrup in a food processor, and spread the cream evenly over the cake bases.

Cover the cakes with foil and place them in the fridge for 2–3 hours.

Garnish, if you wish, with some fresh berries and pieces of dark chocolate.

TIP: You can also make this as 1 large cake in a tin about 20 cm (8 inches) in diameter. If you are in a hurry, put the cake in the freezer. That way it will be ready to eat sooner. When ready to serve, simply cut the cake into small pieces with a pizza cutter.

9

10

11

12

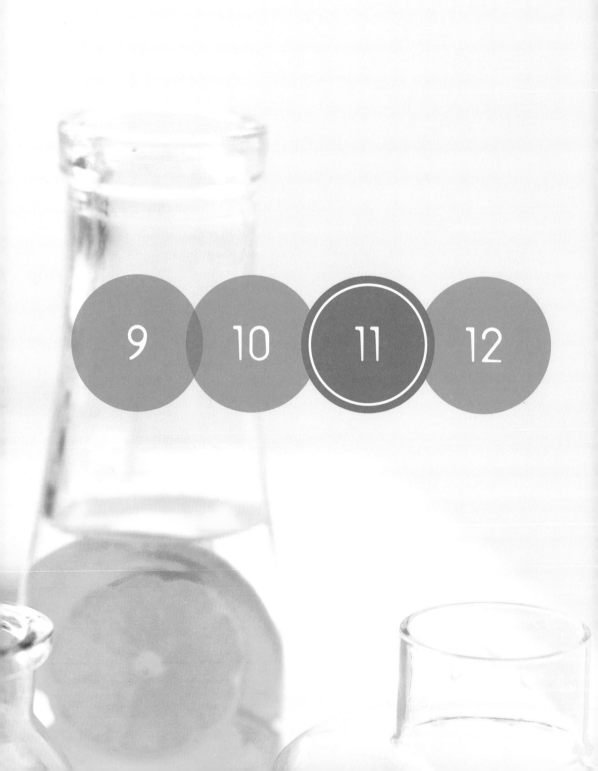

GOAL FOR WEEK 11

This week's exercise may sound the simplest, but it seems to be difficult for many of us – drink water before you feel thirsty, and cut out artificially sweetened drinks. By doing this you will maintain peak metabolism and improve stamina and memory. Without water to drink, even a genius cannot function! When you replace sweetened drinks with free water, you are saving yourself both the cash and the kilos.

DRINK WATER

Improving your metabolism is easier than you think. The positive health benefits of pure water from your own tap are underrated, and many people believe that water is completely free of nutrition. Water is more than just H_2O! It helps out with important minerals, and gives a volume to cells that makes room for complicated processes and vital production. A body containing too little water is like a tent with poles that are too short — nothing much can happen when there's not enough space. Take a few more sips and make space for flawless cell function.

It is a well-known fact that water quenches thirst, but can a glass of water increase weight loss, too? The world's cheapest drink really can help you, in many ways, to reach a stable ideal weight.

By drinking water before mealtimes, you fill up your stomach so that you feel full quicker, and therefore reduce the intake of food. In a study of 48 middle-aged and elderly overweight people, 500 ml (17 fl oz/2 cups) of water given before every main meal produced an extra 2 kg (4 lb 8 oz) of weight loss over 12 weeks, compared to the same diet without water before the food (Dennis 2010). Now, 500 ml sounds a bit much, but if you are able to increase your water consumption to over 1 litre (35 fl oz/ 4 cups) a day, it will also have a significant impact. A study of 173 overweight women on four different diets over 12 months showed that those who drank 1 litre of water or more every day achieved a substantial reduction in weight. They also benefited from increased burning of fat and a slimmer waist than those who drank less water (Stookey 2008). If you drink a 200–300 ml (7–10½ fl oz) glass at all main meals, you have almost guaranteed the effect for yourself.

I have always been bad at drinking water and used to wait until I was so thirsty that I just had to have some. In the mornings I would suffer from headaches and poor concentration at work. Now I always take a large glass of water every time I get myself a cup of coffee, and drink the water before I get another cup of coffee. It works for me, I have fewer headaches and it's easier for me to focus.

When you drink water with a meal, the water travels down to the stomach and dilutes the stomach contents so that the concentration of carbohydrates is lowered. That provides a more balanced blood sugar level, and therefore lower insulin production. This way you avoid the surges in insulin that inhibit your fat burning after mealtimes.

And that's not all – a good balance of fluids combats dehydration in your body, too. When the body is thirsty for water, the cells lose fluid and shrivel a little, in the same way that grapes lose water when they are dried to make raisins. In your cell factories, this shrinkage weakens production, performance and responsiveness. Dehydrated fat cells don't release fatty acids through the bloodstream to the hardworking muscles quite as easily. That results in reduced fat burning (Keller 2003). Fat burning gradually increases as you drink again. Many of us believe that we are drinking enough if we only drink when we are thirsty. When you feel thirsty, your cells are already dehydrated. Even mild dehydration can weaken your physical endurance (Adams 2008). So, always have a bottle of water at the ready and drink a little at regular intervals.

However, it's not just the body and muscles that struggle without enough water. Studies show that dehydration can weaken both your concentration and memory and, furthermore, put a drag on your good mood (Ganio 2011, Armstrong 2012). If you feel a rising brain fog, or are getting irritated, it's not necessarily the fault of low blood sugar. Take a deep breath and fetch yourself a glass of water.

How much water is enough water?

YOU HAVE TO REPLACE LOST FLUIDS BOTH WHEN YOU ARE RESTING AND WHEN YOU ARE ON THE MOVE. WHEN YOU ARE RESTING, FLUID LOSS OCCURS THROUGH THE MOISTURE IN THE AIR THAT YOU BREATHE OUT, FLUID IN THE URINE AND FAECES, AND THROUGH SWEAT. YOU SHOULD REPLACE A RESTING FLUID LOSS OF ABOUT 30 ML (1 FL OZ) PER KILOGRAM OF BODY WEIGHT. THAT MEANS THAT IF YOU WEIGH 70 KG (154 LB), YOU WILL FLOURISH WITH AROUND 2 LITRES (70 FL OZ/ 8 CUPS) OF WATER PER DAY (70 × 30 ML) WHEN RESTING. WHEN YOU ARE MOVING, AND BOTH BREATHING AND SWEATING MORE, THE LOSS OF FLUID INCREASES AND, THEREFORE, ALSO THE NEED TO REPLACE IT.

With moderate physical activity, you should consume 200 ml (7 fl oz) of water from your water bottle every 15 minutes. That's because drier muscles are weaker muscles. If your muscle cells contract because of a lack of water, the breakdown of muscle protein increases (Keller 2003). That means that more water protects you against loss of muscle mass, and that you need less time to build muscle during training. Increased muscle mass means a higher consumption of calories, something that makes it easier for you to keep your weight steady.

It's not just via the water bottle that the body gets its water. You get a little water from fruit, vegetables, tea, soups, and so on. Most people will be well hydrated if they drink around 2 litres (70 fl oz/8 cups) of water daily.

Everything in moderation

DON'T OVERDO YOUR WATER INTAKE! IF YOU DRINK TOO MUCH WATER, IT CAN RESULT IN YOUR BODY FLUIDS BECOMING TOO DILUTED, SOMETHING THAT WORKS AGAINST YOUR METABOLISM. IT WILL SEND YOU ON A CRAZY NUMBER OF TRIPS TO THE BATHROOM, TOO.

9

10

11

12

Switch to calorie-free drinks

You will achieve the most sublime benefits of drinking water by replacing calorie-rich drink products with it. You can save yourself hundreds of calories a day – maybe hundreds of dollars a month, too!

Do you drink half a litre of soft drinks or juice a day? Replacing the bottle of fizz with a bottle of water can save on more than 200 kcal every day. That means that you are sparing yourself around 10 kg (22 lb) of body fat a year. It's clearly easy to drink yourself big.

ARTIFICIALLY SWEET

Many people choose artificially sweetened drinks like diet soft drinks in order to save on calories. Even if they do not contain a single calorie, artificially sweetened drink products nevertheless have a negative influence on body weight. Studies show that these sweet chemicals can actually impair your fat burning. Belly fat cells, especially, seem to be hit hard, so your plan to slim down your waist can be harmed by these types of drinks. In addition, strong sweet flavours may increase sweet cravings, while weakening the sense of satisfaction that sweetness triggers in the brain's pleasure zones, so that you steadily long for sweet tastes (Green 2012).

Some studies now suggest that artificial sweeteners may affect hormones in the intestinal lining, so that they absorb carbohydrates more easily (Brown 2009). In practice this means that such drink products can lead to sugar binges and the increased intake of carbohydrates.

Our knowledge today indicates a possible link between the use of artificial sweeteners and increased body weight in both adults and children (Fowler 2008). Large population studies point towards a connection between the use of artificial sweeteners and the onset of metabolic syndrome and the risk factors for this disease, such as large waist size, high blood pressure and a high blood sugar level when fasting (Nettleton 2009).

Many places around the world have high quality water literally on tap. Stay away from mineral water with artificial sweeteners: flavoured water in the shops can be a cocktail of additives – it's better to flavour your own with natural ingredients and capture the positive health benefits of them. If you want a little freshness and sweetness, add natural sweet flavours using a little honey, sweet herbs and berries or some freshly squeezed juice, lime and lemon. Treat yourself with your homemade flavoured water and carbonated drinks, and enjoy the effect on body and mind.

GOOD ADVICE TO DRINK ENOUGH WATER THROUGHOUT THE DAY

* Choose water as a thirst quencher.

* Consider drinking water at room temperature – some people find that they drink more when it's not freezing cold.

* Have a bottle of water at hand, in your purse or bag.

* Always take a bottle of water with you when you go out for a walk.

* Put a water bottle by your computer. Take a sip every time you lift your head and your mind starts to drift.

* Drink a glass of water between cups of coffee. That means that you fill up the cup and the glass at the same time and don't go to fetch another coffee before the glass of water is empty.

* Take a bottle of water with you into meetings.

* Fill up a large jug with soda water, flavoured if you prefer, and have it to hand when you are watching TV or reading a book. Buy pure soda water or make it yourself. Soda water machines are not expensive.

* Make iced tea from green tea (see page 224) in the evening and put it in the fridge before you go to bed. That way you have a drink ready for the next day that also counts as water!

* Make bottles of flavoured water (see page 239) in advance and place them in the fridge. Leave them to cool for several hours so that the flavours infuse in the water. Try using slices of cucumber, orange or raspberries.

9

10

11

12

Now you have not just replaced calorie-rich drink products with water and increased your water intake, you have also made it easier for yourself to build muscle mass and burn fat. Every single sip of pure water helps along the road to a slimmer waist and a greater joy in life, better health and more energy. This is a tool that you can even get for free, straight from your own tap – the simplest way is often the best.

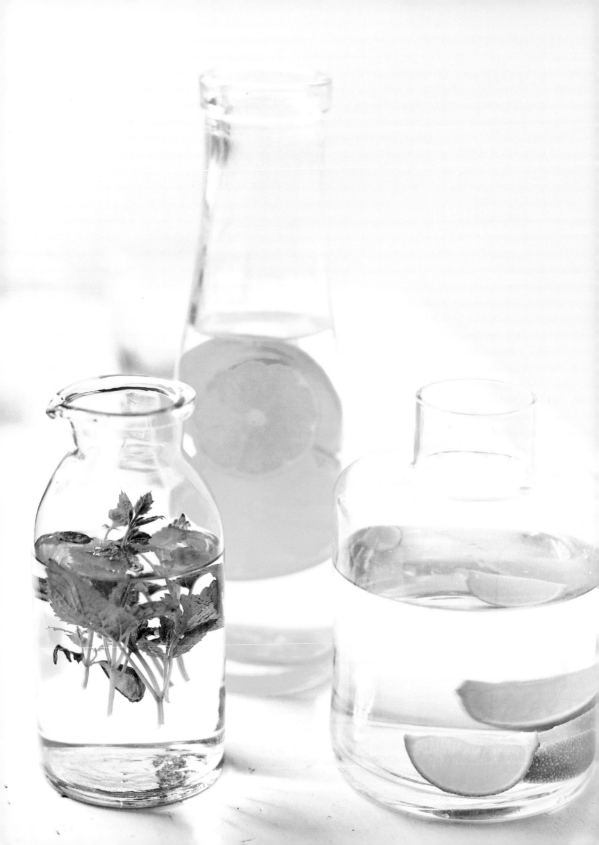

Flavoured water

Fill up a glass bottle or a carafe with pure water and add your favourite flavours.

The small bottle in the photograph has fresh mint in it. The tall bottle contains slices of organic orange, and the small carafe has lime wedges.
Wash the herbs and citrus fruits well before using them.
Put the bottle in the fridge and drink 1 litre (35 fl oz/4 cups) throughout the day.

9

10

11

12

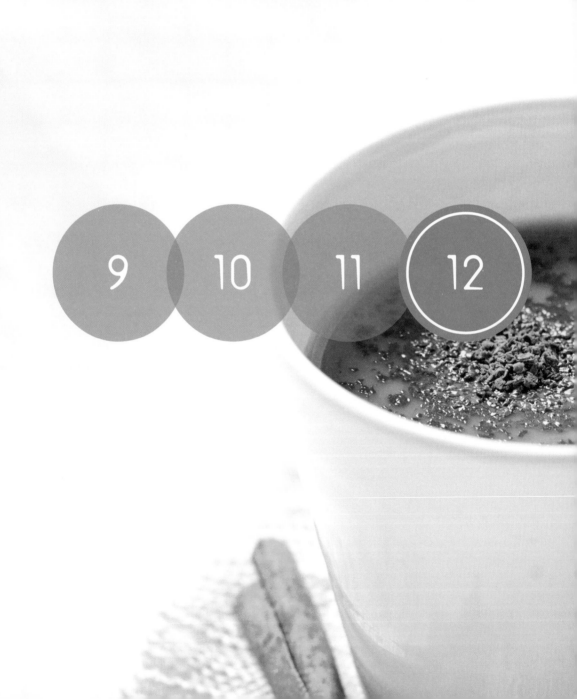

GOAL FOR WEEK 12

This week's exercise is to understand and use the method so that it leads to lasting changes to your daily diet. In order to nurture lasting change, this week you are getting many delicacies you can enjoy. The method's final weekly task offers desserts, cosy drinks and snacks that look like treats but count as 'vegetables'. They stave off persistent cravings, boost your health, increase your quality of life and help you to achieve a stable weight – it's all about enjoyment, because you deserve the very best!

TREAT YOURSELF TO SMART SNACKS

Even if this book is drawing to a close, it's just the beginning for you. It's the start of the rest of your life. Over the course of a few weeks you have succeeded in changing habits in a way that will have vital significance for your life ahead. This week's advice on smart snacks is the finishing touch, and demonstrates that the method is filled with pleasure, not sacrifice. Treat yourself to some delicious snacks that look like dessert, but count as vegetables. Enjoy great flavours that increase fat burning and set the scene, in the best possible way, for the good life.

Good in-between meals can keep your metabolism up, a little bit like adding a log to the fire to keep the embers alive. The wrong type of snack food can, however, upset your metabolism by triggering sugar cravings and overeating.

The difference lies in whether you choose pure foods with nutrients that your body needs, or heavily processed foods and quick carbohydrates to obtain seemingly instant gratification.

In a nutshell: you have to fuel your fire at the right time and in the right way, so that the body achieves the best metabolism it can while you enjoy an even heat from the billions of glowing cells.

Keep nuts, seeds and water to hand

Chocolate bars, hard sweets, biscuits and buns are not good fuel. They're like throwing paper on the fire – paper burns up at the speed of lightning, leaving behind nothing but ashes that can choke the embers. Choosing these kinds of quick carbs also triggers blood sugar alarms in your body, so that you find yourself in an ever-growing battle against sugar cravings. Maybe you are struggling to break out of a vicious cycle: the snacks you choose to satisfy the cravings just make everything worse. It's easily done – a small biscuit quickly turns into the whole packet, or the chocolate bar vanishes even though you only planned to take a little nibble. It is difficult and challenging to manage a sugar craving, so here I suggest snack choices that can keep it at bay. Read more about sugar cravings on page 22.

With nuts and seeds in your diet you avoid alarmingly high blood sugar peaks, stress hormones and insulin surges – and a body that struggles with sickness and low energy. Choose treats and snacks that fill the body with energy, and free yourself from the eternal fight against the vicious cycle. In addition to quick carbohydrates, ready-made snacks contain a cocktail of unnecessary ingredients – everything from hydrogenated fats to artificial E-numbers. Many packets of biscuits feature a long list of ingredients that, at best, have no possible benefit for you … and, at worst, are actually harmful to your health. If you choose junk food only occasionally, this will probably not affect your health. However, a daily intake may contribute towards both poor health and a larger waist. It is what you eat every day that has the biggest health effects.

The situation is not made any easier by the way we surround ourselves, at all times, with food. Photos of convenient food choices catch the eye and trigger cravings constantly. When you are filling up with petrol, you are met by a '3 for 2' offer on pastries; when you are buying coffee, you get a free muffin; and when you are at the movies, a trip to the candy bar for chocolate and popcorn is promoted as an essential part of the experience. It is more important than ever for you to keep your blood sugar and hunger hormones in check, so you can free yourself from the craving's claws, and take control. Here you will not only get tools that help you to resist those temptations, but also knowledge that really changes your needs and desires – once you let yourself be enticed by smart snack choices.

9

10

11

12

There are two tools that can especially help you to win this fight: the first is to keep cravings at a distance; the second is knowledge about snacks that do you good. These tools make it possible to hush the hunger hormones' screaming for empty calories, and to let yourself feel the euphoria that occurs when the body is filled with spirit and energy from natural sweetness and protein-rich food.

Most of us probably recognise the hunger hormones' cry as an all-consuming desire for a particular type of food – often something that you know will do you no good. If you are sick of the struggle against your own appetite, the solution is not to resist all snacks and evening treats. It's like holding your breath – sooner or later, you will have to exhale. When your brain is focused on *avoiding* food, your desire for it is stronger than ever. No matter how many sticks of carrot you munch, the craving will not disappear.

But that doesn't mean that the only answer is giving in. You can prevent sugar cravings and teach yourself smart tricks so you can take control as soon as the munchies start. The idea is to plan snacks and evening treats that you can look forward to and that the mind and body can enjoy – mini-meals that keep your blood sugar stable, your hunger hormones at bay, and troublesome cravings away. These little meals should consist of protein, fibre, low glycaemic index (GI) carbohydrates, plant nutrients and healthy fatty acids in order to be able to satisfy hunger in the best possible way. This kind of food is slowly digested, consumes energy, guarantees stable blood sugar and keeps cravings cornered. As an addition to your three main meals, these snacks can actually increase your metabolism and contribute towards better weight loss (Conceição de Oliveira 2003).

YOU ARE DOING THE BODY – AND THE WAISTLINE – A BIG FAVOUR IF YOU AVOID:

1 Biscuits and cakes (a lot of sugar, wheat flour and unhealthy fat)
2 Energy bars (which provide a lot of energy – and therefore calories – but few well-preserved nutrients)
3 Salty snacks like potato chips and salted nuts

TIPS FOR SMARTER SNACK CHOICES IN DAILY LIFE

* Plan in-between meals and snacks (prevents sugar cravings from being triggered).

* Keep an eye on portion size (a small box with a handful of nuts per day).

* Combine sweet fruit with proteins and fats in order to avoid triggering the blood sugar alarm and sugar cravings (for example, yoghurt and cottage cheese with half a sliced banana instead of a whole banana alone, or a thin layer of organic peanut butter spread on half a banana – the peanut butter must be organic).

GREAT ADVICE FOR WHEN SUGAR CRAVINGS GO WILD

* Munch 5–6 nuts at a time, not a whole handful. Take your time and chew well. The chewing and the great taste will satisfy you. Drink water (200–300 ml/7–10½ fl oz), or have a cup of green tea. Ten minutes later the craving will have vanished!

* Try to change your focus. Perform an action that forces the brain to think of something else for 10 minutes. One of my patients thinks that it helps to do the opposite of what she had just been doing. If you are sitting, stand up. If you are inside, put your coat on and go out. When the brain is occupied by solving other issues, sugar cravings are pushed to the back of the mind.

* If these tips aren't helping, take a little piece of dark chocolate and treat yourself to a cup of coffee.

9

10

11

12

Take note of what works for
you – we are all different!

ENCOURAGE REST WHILE YOU SLEEP

MANY BELIEVE THAT WHEN WE SLEEP, WE PUT ON WEIGHT MORE EASILY BECAUSE THE METABOLISM GOES TO SLEEP WHEN WE DO. THIS IS ONLY PARTIALLY TRUE. IT MAY BE EASIER TO OVEREAT IN THE EVENING BECAUSE YOUR BODY DOESN'T PRODUCE THE FULLNESS HORMONES QUITE AS EASILY AT THAT TIME OF THE DAY. THE CALORIES ARE BURNED AS ENERGY, HOWEVER, AND THE NUTRIENTS ARE USED FOR GROWTH AND REPAIR.

YOUR EVENING MEALS SHOULD THEREFORE HELP YOU TO GET THE BEST POSSIBLE REST. IT MAKES SENSE TO EAT A SMALL EVENING MEAL WITH NATURAL CARBOHYDRATES THAT PROMOTE A GOOD NIGHT'S SLEEP BY INCREASING THE PRODUCTION OF MELATONIN, THE SLEEP HORMONE. GETTING ENOUGH SLEEP ACTUALLY MAKES IT EASIER FOR YOU TO ACHIEVE A STABLE IDEAL WEIGHT.

Snacks and a good night's sleep

Did you know that your sleep at night and your daily cycles have an effect on how you register hunger and fullness? Lack of sleep is doubly bad in the context of weight, because it increases the sensation of hunger and dulls the feeling of fullness when you over-eat. So, have you ever been told to sleep more if you want to lose weight? Now you know that sleep really can help towards a slimmer waist. Sleep deficiency increases the production of ghrelin, the hunger hormone, which increases the appetite and interferes with fat burning. The less sleep you get, the harder your body holds on to its belly fat.

Sleep more – burn more: A German study from the University of Lübeck, in which the participants were kept awake all night, measured a drop of 5% in the resting metabolism and a total drop of 20% in energy burning after meals, relative to energy burning after a good night's sleep (Schmid 2008).

Sleep more – curb cravings: A lack of sleep lowers the levels of leptin, the hormone that makes you feel full. An American study showed that participants who were woken after 5½ hours of sleep snacked 50% more between mealtimes the next day, relative to when they slept 2½ hours more (Nedeltcheva 2009).

Give yourself 7–9 hours of quality sleep every night. It is a myth that you can catch up on lost sleep by snoozing through the whole weekend. It is important to take time to relax before you sleep. If you can, go to bed an hour earlier, and read until you become tired. Make sure that the bedroom is dark, cool and airy. Even the light from a clock radio can reduce the quality of your sleep. Use blackout curtains and turn the clock face away from you.

9

10

11

12

PLANT POWER INCREASES FAT BURNING

More new research reports are emerging showing that nature's plant power works wonders for your body. Fat burning is no exception!

What you eat can create the conditions for the effective reading of the cells' gene codes, optimal maintenance, suitable production and appropriate metabolism. On the other hand, your food choices can lead to blood sugar chaos, lower energy and a greater storage of fat.

Some plant nutrients can help you to achieve a slimmer waist in an effective way by making you feel full more easily, and they can make sure that you don't easily store fat around your middle. They can do that by increasing the sensitivity of the cells' receptors, so they can more easily receive signals from hormones and neurotransmitters. Furthermore, that means that both insulin and the fullness hormone function better, which gives you all the benefits mentioned above.

When your cells need to produce something, they find the code in your genes. The plant nutrients affect which gene codes in your cells are read; this is expressed in the form of cell products like new receptors, neurotransmitters and hormones. Particular gene codes, called sirtuins, are given priority when you eat more plant nutrients. Think of them as the doormen. Sirtuins decide which codes will be read and which ones will be skipped over. Having more doormen means that more gene codes are read to create new receptors or antennae on the surface of the cell. More antennae means increased sensitivity of the cells to signals from insulin, and substances that make you feel fresh and happy.

Both stress and poor diet can intensify the assault from fierce inflammatory substances, at the same time as *reducing* the level of sirtuins in your cells. Many types of plant nutrients can curb the inflammatory chaos while strengthening sirtuin's protectiveness! Many plant nutrients can probably take the credit – maybe even more than we have yet discovered. Studies have proven the effects of the polyphenols resveratrol and quercetin, which you can easily get from colourful berries, some grapes, some raw peanuts and a splash of red wine.

Plants and berries form polyphenols when they are damaged – by being stepped on, by sunlight or by being attacked by fungi. The polyphenols repair the damage to the plants and if you choose to eat those plants, the power of polyphenols in them will also protect your cells (Lekli 2010, Chong 2012).

The power of polyphenols can defend you against a range of health problems, prevent cancer, slow down the ageing process, and increase your lifespan by protecting you against the chaos of inflammation and by strengthening the quality controls within your cells. The polyphenol resveratrol seems to come out on top, and has shown itself to enhance the reading of many protective genes that are known to have a connection to long life (for example, SirT1, FoxO, PBEF). Some of the plant nutrients don't even need to be absorbed in the intestine in any significant quantity in order to take effect. Some work with helpful bacteria in the gut; others heal a weakened intestinal lining; while others still are absorbed into every single cell in the body. The rebuilding and activation of plant nutrients by the bacterial helpers in the intestine can be the key to triggering their positive health benefits (Walle 2011). We don't know the full story about this relationship yet, but while we wait for even more insights, we can simply enjoy the wondrous power of plants.

Even if all the workings are not fully understood yet, polyphenol-rich food seems to strengthen the cells' quality controls (Lekli 2010). The common feature in grapes and berries is that they increase the number of doormen in the cells, improving insulin sensitivity, reducing the demand for insulin production and cutting down belly fat.

Resveratrol steers the cells in your belly fat towards preparation for fatty acids and enhanced fat burning. When, for different reasons, cells are drowning in fat, they react by protecting themselves – a survival technique. They produce a protein miracle cure called adiponectin, which has characteristics that hinder fat, diabetes and inflammation (Ma 2009). Together, resveratrol and adiponectin help to increase the metabolism of fatty acids, improve cholesterol levels, boost insulin sensitivity, correct blood pressure, restrict inflammation and defend against sickness (dos Santos Costa 2011).

The polyphenol quercetin boasts similar virtues. Quercetin in onions, green vegetables, parsley, apple peel, berries, citrus fruit, tea and red wine can decrease inflammation and oxidative stress, lower blood pressure, reduce the amount of triglycerides and bad cholesterol, boost insulin sensitivity, raise the level of protective adiponectin in the belly fat cells, intensify fat burning and diminish the storage of fat in the liver and around the waist.

It is fantastic that different plants can play their part with your belly fat cells, taking up the fight against an expanding waist and thwarting sickness. So feast on these valuable plant foods, full of wonderful, natural flavours and lots of smart nutrients per calorie – and let these plant-powered treats work their magic on your health.

Don't blindly believe that a snack bar is healthy just because it says 'healthy, protein, low carb' on the label. The perfect snack is a mini-meal of nature's own treasures – it doesn't need a declaration of ingredients.

Empty the pantry and fridge of sweets, salty snacks, biscuits, cakes and soft drinks. Replace them with ingredients for smart snacks. Always be prepared by restocking the cupboards and fridge with smart snack choices.

9

10

11

12

WHAT TO HAVE IN THE PANTRY AND FRIDGE FOR MAKING SMART SNACKS

* Low glycaemic index (GI) fruit (such as apples, pears, plums and nectarines)

* Fibre-rich fruit (apples, kiwi fruit, grapefruit)

* All types of berries – fresh and frozen

* Various unsalted nuts and seeds, such as almonds, cashew nuts, walnuts, Brazil nuts, pepitas (pumpkin seeds) and sesame seeds

* Ingredients for hummus: chickpeas, tahini, garlic, olive oil

* Organic peanut butter

* Cottage cheese, plain yoghurt and buttermilk

* Blue cheese

* Avocados, tomatoes, onion, garlic and chilli for guacamole

* Snack vegetables such as carrots, celery stalks and cucumber – cut them up, lay them on a plate and sprinkle a little chilli powder over them

* Pure (not processed) meat like turkey, chicken, roast beef, lamb, ham and other beef cuts that you can slice up and keep in a box in the fridge

* Green salad leaves and kale for kale chips

* Green tea in different flavours

* Dates and figs

* Sardines, herrings or anchovies and chopped red onion to serve on small crackers

* Eggs

TIPS FOR SMART SNACK CHOICES

* 200 g (7 oz) chopped fruit or fresh berries mixed with 100 g (3½ oz) plain yoghurt and 1 tablespoon cottage cheese; sprinkle 5–10 chopped nuts on top

* 2 tablespoons guacamole dip and vegetable spears with chilli spices (page 149) plus 50 g (1¾ oz) thinly sliced fresh deli meat

* 2 tablespoons hummus, vegetable spears plus 30–50 g (1–1¾ oz) thinly sliced deli meat

* Smoked salmon slices with 1 teaspoon cream cheese, herbs (chives, flat-leaf parsley) and chopped red onion wrapped in a cabbage leaf or a strong lettuce leaf

* Spiced or cured herring with 1 teaspoon sour cream, red onion and flat-leaf parsley (plus ½ slice rye bread)

* 5–10 nuts plus 2 dates plus a little bit of ground cinnamon blended together using a stick blender; roll it up into a ball, press flat on to a plate and top with 1 tablespoon Greek-style yoghurt, fresh berries and kiwi fruit

* Green salad with 2 handfuls assorted salad leaves, 2 tablespoons avocado, 1 hard-boiled egg in segments or fish/meat leftovers plus 1 tablespoon French vinaigrette (page 187)

* Celery stalks filled with a little nut butter, cream cheese or blue cheese

* Powderless protein smoothie (page 163)

* Green wraps (page 73)

* 100 g (3½ oz) plain yoghurt, 2 tablespoons Berit's breakfast cereal (page 55) or quick rolled (porridge) oats, and the seeds from ½ pomegranate

* Raspberry gratin (page 259)

* 1 sliced apple with ½ teaspoon ground cinnamon and 5 chopped pecans roasted in the oven; serve with 100 g (3½ oz) plain yoghurt

* Popcorn popped in coconut oil or extra virgin olive oil at a moderate temperature

* A bowl of porridge with 100 g (3½ oz) blueberries and 1 tablespoon Greek-style yoghurt

* A small bowl of barley porridge with ½ apple, chopped into pieces, and ½ teaspoon ground cinnamon

* Oven-baked egg avocado (page 189)

9

10

11

12

Be prepared for when cravings strike by having chopped and portioned treats ready for the day. Make a few smart snacks that you can put into containers and store in the fridge ahead of time. By planning your treats, you will find that you take control of your appetite. Use your energy on what you enjoy, not what you need to avoid – then you have an unbeatable plan, and the desire for unhealthy snacks will disappear, along with your stomach fat. You really deserve congratulations and praise now that you have put 12 demanding weeks behind you. Hopefully it has been an exciting time that has provided fantastic results. Some are measurable and visible; others can only be enjoyed by thinking of what you have achieved for the rest of your life – better health and vitality! Congratulations on your choice – now you have laid the groundwork to be able to enjoy every single memorable moment. Keep in mind: it is not happy *days* that stick in the mind, but happy *moments*. Before you put this book down for the last time, you have already extended your life expectancy by several years of those moments – so all that remains is to make them memorable!

NOT ALL CALORIES ARE CREATED EQUAL. LET THE FRUITS OF THE GARDEN OF EDEN TEMPT YOU, WITH SMART CALORIES FROM REAL FOOD. INDULGE IN REAL FOOD FOR A BETTER LIFE – BECAUSE YOU OWE YOURSELF THE BEST!

The food that you eat is not made up of just calories, but also of nutrients that build up the mind and body and that program your cells. Over the course of 12 weeks you have been able to take on valuable knowledge from advanced medical research. You have received insights into ingredients that set up the body for better health, greater happiness and more energy. You have learned how to listen to your own needs, you live more in harmony with your body's desires, and you benefit from food choices that improve your mood and your waist size, so your mind and body can both shine. In a short space of time you have replaced food that strangles vitality and motivation with food that creates good health and a new drive. You are enjoying foods that program you for energy and pleasure. Your choice is good for the environment and lays the best foundations for a wonderful life. You have made a fantastic effort, so enjoy the result – because you deserve it!

PLEASE SHARE YOUR KNOWLEDGE AND EXPERIENCE – TOGETHER WE CAN MAKE A DIFFERENCE!

9

10

11

12

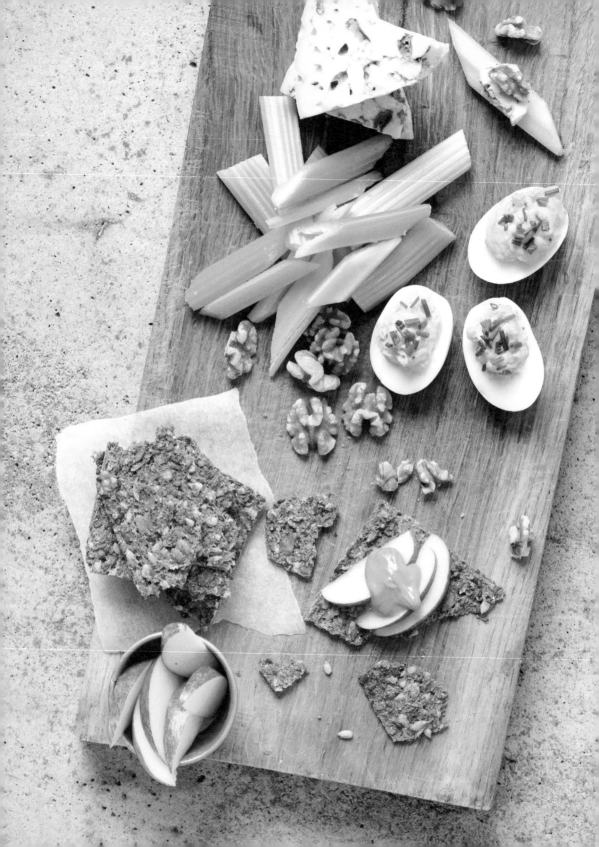

Finger food

CELERY STALKS WITH BLUE CHEESE AND WALNUTS

GLUTEN-FREE CRACKERS (PAGE 57) WITH APPLES AND ORGANIC PEANUT BUTTER FOR DIP

DEVILLED EGGS
6 hard-boiled eggs
3 tablespoons mayonnaise
1 tablespoon mustard
sea salt and freshly ground black pepper
fresh herbs, such as chives and flat-leaf (Italian) parsley, to garnish

Cut the eggs in half lengthwise. Remove the yolks.
Mash the egg yolks, mayonnaise, mustard, salt and pepper to a creamy consistency.
Fill the egg halves with the cream. Garnish with the herbs.

TIP: Use your favourite mustard – I think wholegrain mustard tastes really good in this recipe.

9

10

11

12

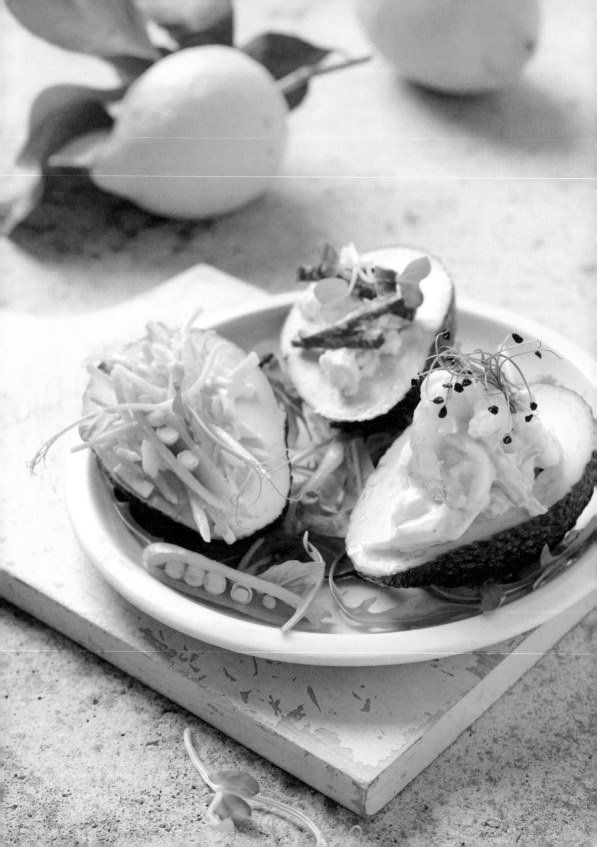

Avocado with different fillings

A ripe avocado is a gift to all those who love good food. Cut it in half, remove the stone and enjoy the flesh with a little extra virgin olive oil, freshly ground black pepper, some sea salt and a few drops of lemon juice. If you want to make an appetiser from avocados, the possibilities are endless.

PRAWNS AND MAYONNAISE
5–6 cooked peeled prawns (shrimp)
2 teaspoons mayonnaise
1 teaspoon lemon juice
sea salt and freshly ground black pepper

FETA AND HAM
1 tablespoon crumbled feta cheese
small strips of ham or other cured meat

RAW VEGETABLES
1 tablespoon finely grated carrot and cabbage
2 teaspoons mayonnaise
sea salt and freshly ground black pepper

TO GARNISH
sea salt and freshly ground black pepper
lemon juice
fresh herbs, such as chives and flat-leaf (Italian) parsley

Combine the ingredients for your chosen filling.
Cut the avocado in half and remove the stone, then spoon in your chosen filling. Sprinkle over some grains of salt and a little pepper, a few drops of lemon juice and something green to top it off – for example, some chives, flat-leaf parsley or other green herbs.

9

10

11

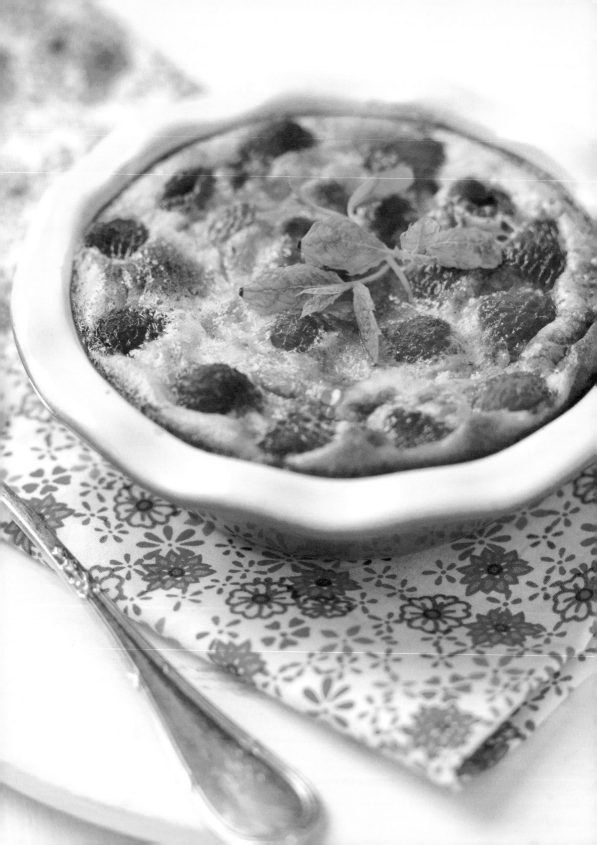

Raspberry gratin

This simple dessert provides lots of nutrition from eggs and berries, at the same time as warming the heart.

SERVES 2

200 g (7 oz) frozen raspberries or whatever berries you have in the house
2 eggs
1–2 tablespoons honey
mint, to garnish

Preheat the oven to 200°C (400°F).
Put the raspberries in an ovenproof dish.
Whisk the eggs and honey until they are light and fluffy. Pour the egg mixture over the raspberries.
Bake the gratin in the oven for 5–6 minutes. Serve topped with a sprig of mint.

9

10

11

12

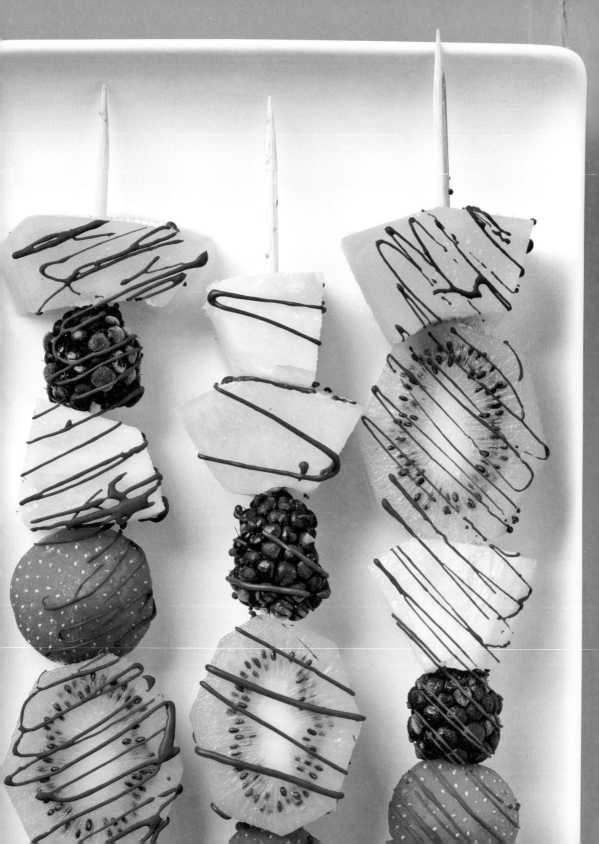

Fruit skewers with chocolate

This is a totally brilliant way to get children of all ages to eat a healthy dessert full of beneficial nutrients. Choose fruit and berries that the kids especially love. Here are some suggestions:

kiwi fruit
pineapple
strawberries
rockmelon
blackberries

CHOCOLATE DRIZZLE
dark chocolate (80% cocoa solids)

Cut the fruit into pieces and thread the fruit onto wooden skewers.
Put the skewers in the freezer for at least 1 hour.
Melt the chocolate in a heatproof bowl set over a saucepan of simmering water.
Drizzle the melted chocolate over the fruit, and refrigerate until set. Enjoy!

9

10

11

12

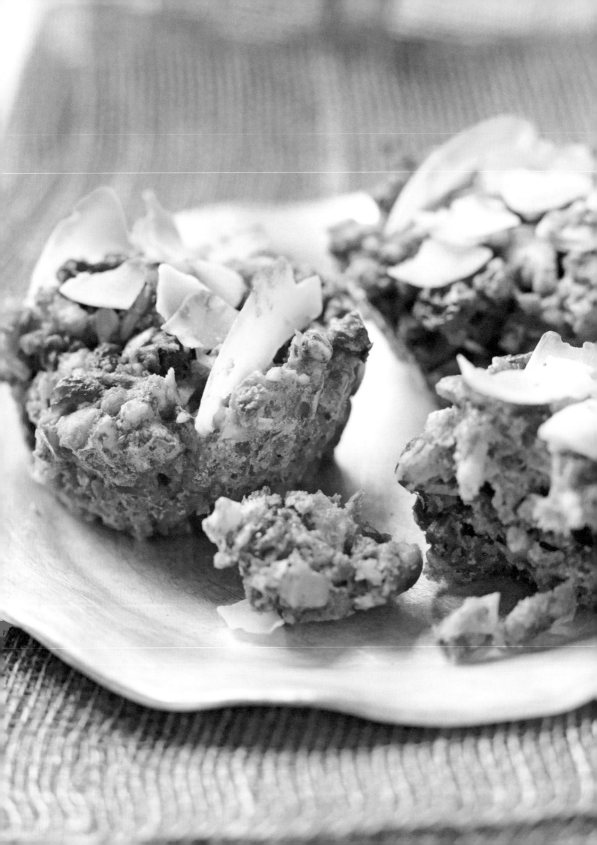

Nut temptations

These lovely nut cakes taste great with coffee at home, but are also really nice to take on a walk. They give you just enough energy to manage the last long climb of a Sunday stroll.

MAKES 10–12 SMALL CAKES

250 g (9 oz) walnuts or pecans
125 g (4½ oz) sunflower seeds
125 g (4½ oz) raisins
2 tablespoons coconut flour or grated coconut
2 teaspoons ground cinnamon
¼ teaspoon sea salt
1 banana
2 tablespoons linseeds (flaxseeds)
2 tablespoons apple juice
1 tablespoon melted organic extra virgin coconut oil
1 tablespoon honey
toasted coconut flakes, to garnish

Preheat the oven to 175°C (350°F).
Fill a 12-hole muffin tray with paper cases.
Chop the nuts and mix with the sunflower seeds, raisins, coconut, cinnamon and sea salt in a bowl.
Mash the banana, and grind the linseeds quickly in a blender so that they are lightly crushed.
Mix the banana, linseeds, apple juice, coconut oil and honey together in another bowl.
Pour the banana mixture into the bowl with the nuts and seeds, and mix well. Divide the dough among the muffin cups, pressing it down firmly.
Bake the cakes in the centre of the preheated oven for 20 minutes. Leave them to cool on a cooling rack. Garnish with toasted coconut flakes before serving.
Store the cakes in an airtight container where they'll keep for up to 2 weeks.

9
10
11
12

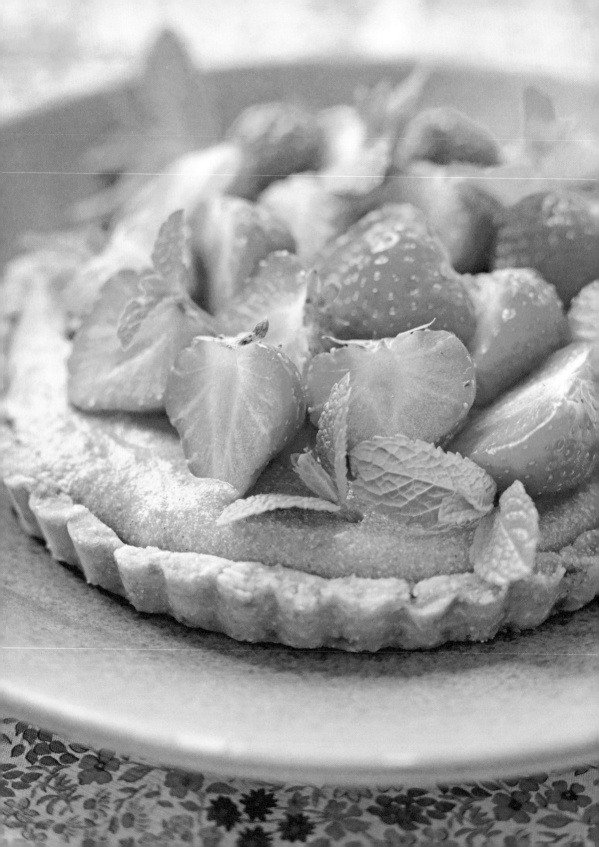

Totally raw strawberry tart

This is a fantastically fresh dessert that is simple to make – preferably a few days before it will be eaten.

SERVES 4–5

sliced banana or strawberries (optional)
strawberries, halved, to garnish
1 small handful mint leaves, to garnish

TART BASE
1 banana
150 g (5½ oz/1½ cups) rolled (porridge) oats
150 g (5½ oz/1½ cups) almond meal or almond flour
pinch of sea salt
coconut oil, for greasing

STRAWBERRY CREAM
6–7 dates
10–12 strawberries
4 tablespoons melted organic extra virgin coconut butter
¼ teaspoon vanilla seeds
¼ teaspoon sea salt
1 tablespoon freshly squeezed lemon juice

To make the base, mash the banana, and mix in the rolled oats, almond meal and sea salt. Knead to a smooth dough.
Grease an 18 cm (7 inch) diameter tart tin with the coconut oil. Press out the dough into the base of the tin and a little over the edge. Cover with plastic wrap and place in the fridge.
To make the strawberry cream, start by removing the stones from the dates and chopping them finely. Mix all the ingredients for the cream in a blender at full speed for 2 minutes, until you have a smooth cream.
Cover the tart base with the banana and strawberry slices, if using, and pour the cream on top. Place the tart in the fridge for a few hours or overnight. It can also be frozen.
When ready to serve, top with fresh strawberries and mint leaves.

9

10

11

12

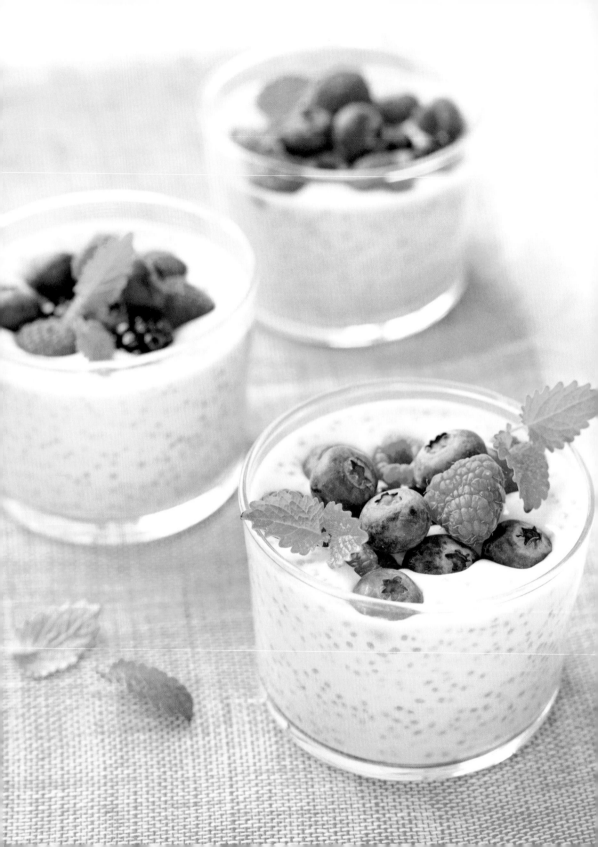

Chia pudding

Omega-3 rich chia seeds are perfect for puddings, and puddings are perfect for dessert. Enjoy!

SERVES 4

350 ml (12 fl oz) reduced-fat coconut milk
2 tablespoons honey
½ teaspoon vanilla seeds
½ teaspoon almond extract
100 g (3½ oz) chia seeds
1 handful colourful berries, to garnish
mint or lemon balm leaves, to garnish

Whisk together the coconut milk, honey, vanilla seeds and almond extract. Stir in the chia seeds. Divide the mixture between 4 dessert glasses, cover and refrigerate for at least 1 hour until set. Take the glasses out of the fridge 15 minutes before serving so that they reach room temperature. The puddings are best eaten the day they are made. Serve topped with berries and mint or lemon balm leaves.

TIP: Use reduced-fat coconut milk, or at least avoid using the white layer of fat in the carton or tin.

9

10

11

12

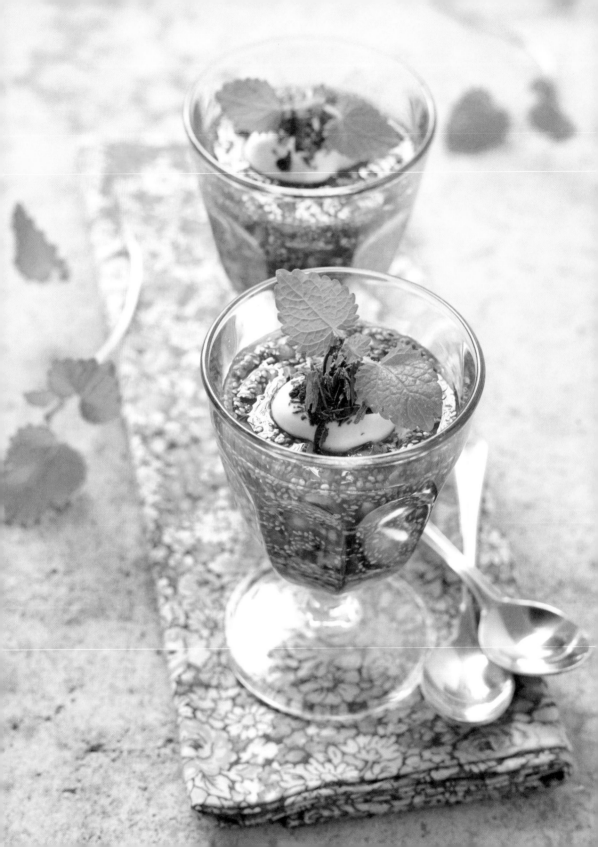

Pomegranate parfait

SERVES 4

1 large pomegranate
3 tablespoons chia seeds
2 tablespoons honey
150 ml (5 fl oz) pomegranate juice or apple juice
1 tablespoon freshly squeezed lemon juice
4 tablespoons plain yoghurt
grated dark chocolate, to garnish
lemon balm leaves, to garnish

Squeeze the pomegranate a little, and cut it in half. Turn each half inside out and scrape out the seeds.

Put the pomegranate seeds, chia seeds, honey, pomegranate juice and lemon juice in a bowl, and stir well.

Divide the mixture among 4 dessert glasses. Cover them with plastic wrap and place them in the fridge for 2–3 hours.

When ready to serve, top the pomegranate parfaits with the yoghurt, and garnish with a little grated dark chocolate and lemon balm leaves.

9

10

11

12

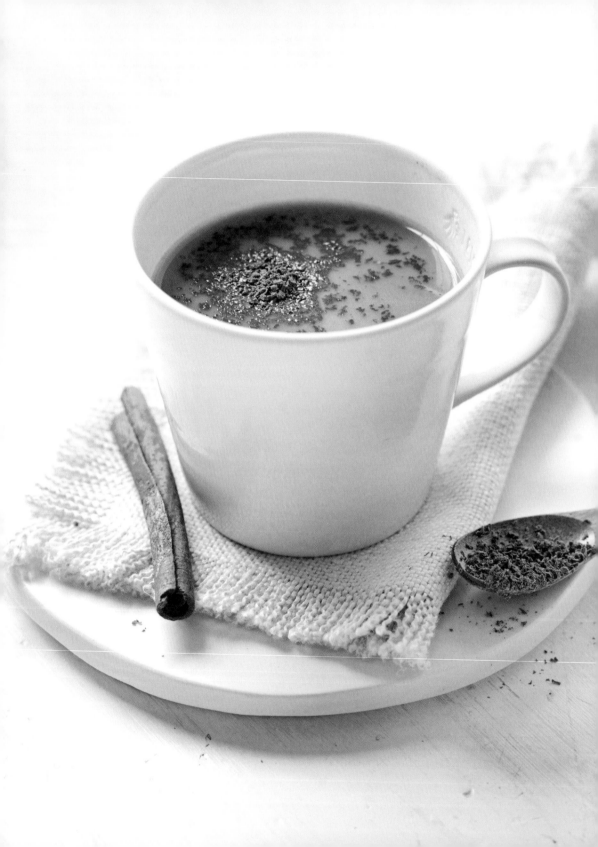

Dessert coffee for two

SERVES 2

200 ml (7 fl oz) milk
300 ml (10½ fl oz) strong coffee
1 teaspoon ground cinnamon
1 teaspoon cocoa
1 teaspoon honey

Note: To make the coffee, coarsely grind your own coffee beans, and make some strong plunger coffee.

Steam the milk with a small, handheld milk steamer.
Pour the steamed milk into two large cups. Pour in the coffee. Stir in the cinnamon and cocoa with a fork.
Divide the honey between two spoons. Place each one in its cup, stir and serve.

9

10

11

12

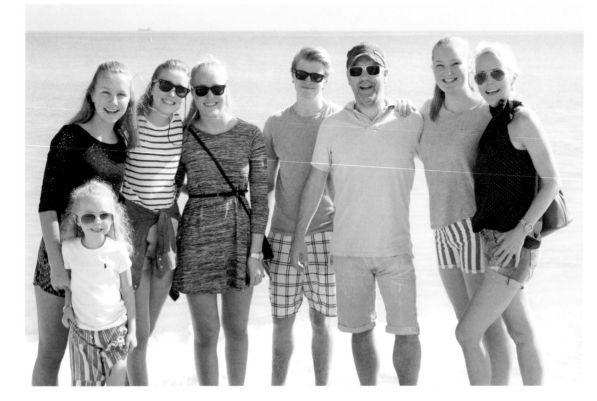

THANKS

A warm thanks to my children and to my husband for showing patience and understanding when I have used days as well as hours late into the evening to produce a book that can improve the quality of life for so very many. In addition, I thank the creative and enthusiastic photographers and employees at Studio Dreyer Hensley, Nina, Jim, Hanne and Thea. Last, but no means least, I want to thank Lars Røtterud at Gyldendal for taking the initiative with the book, for his professional help, fantastic support and inspiration all the way. I am so sincerely happy that I have been able to collaborate with so many talented people – together we have created a book that can help as many people as possible to enjoy the best version of themselves – because they deserve it!

REFERENCES

Introduction

- de Onis et al 2010. Global prevalence and trends of overweight and obesity among preschool children. *The American journal of clinical nutrition*, 92(5), p. 1257–1264.
- Magarey AM, Daniels LA & Boulton TJC 2001. Prevalence of overweight and obesity in Australian children and adolescents: reassessment of 1985 and 1995 data against new standard international definitions. *Medical Journal of Australia* 174:561–4.
- NZ Ministry of Health 2015. Annual Update of Key Results 2014/15: New Zealand Health Survey.
- Australian Bureau of Statistics 2005. National Health Survey 2004–05: Summary of results. ABS cat.no. 4364.0. Canberra: ABS.

Week 1

- Bogdanov S et al 2008. Honey for nutrition and health: a review. *Journal of the American College of Nutrition* 27(6): p. 677–689.
- van Can JGP et al 2009. Reduced glycaemic and insulinaemic responses following isomaltulose ingestion: implications for postprandial substrate use. *British Journal of Nutrition* 102(10), p. 1408.
- Yaghoobi N et al 2008. Natural honey and cardiovascular risk factors; effects on blood glucose, cholesterol, triacylglycerole, CRP, and body weight compared with sucrose. *The Scientific World Journal* 8, p. 463–469.
- Brown CM et al 2008. Sugary drinks in the pathogenesis of obesity and cardiovascular diseases. *International Journal of Obesity* 32, p. 28–34.
- Collinson KS et al 2010. Sugar-sweetened carbonated beverage consumption correlates with BMI, waist circumference, and poor dietary choices in school children. *BMC public health* 10(1), p. 234.

Week 2

- Wycherley TP et al 2010. A high-protein diet with resistance exercise training improves weight loss and body composition in overweight and obese patients with type 2 diabetes. *Diabetes Care* 33(5), p. 969–976.
- Kelesidis IT et al 2006. Adiponectin and cancer: a systematic review. *British Journal of Cancer* 94(9): p. 1221–1225.
- Qi L et al 2006. Dietary fibres and glycaemic load, obesity, and plasma adiponectin levels in women with type 2 diabetes. *Diabetes Care* 29(7), p. 1501–1505.

Week 3

- Wu X et al 2004. Lipophilic and Hydrophilic Antioxidant Capacities of Common Foods in the United States. *Journal of Agricultural and Food Chemistry* 52(12), p. 4026–4037.
- Mizuno CS 2013. Blueberries and Metabolic Syndrome. *Silpakorn University Science and Technology Journal* 3(2), p. 7–17.
- Davis JN et al 2009. Inverse relation between dietary fibre intake and visceral adiposity in overweight Latino youth. *The American journal of clinical nutrition* 90(5), p. 1160–1166.
- Karhunen LJ et al 2010. A psyllium fibre-enriched meal strongly attenuates postprandial gastrointestinal peptide release in healthy young adults. *The Journal of nutrition* 140(4), p. 737–744.
- Howarth, NC et al 2001. Dietary fibre and weight regulation. *Nutrition reviews* 59(5), p. 129–139.
- Johnston KL et al 2010. Resistant starch improves insulin sensitivity in metabolic syndrome. *Diabetic Medicine* 27(4), p. 391–397.
- Alinia SOH et al 2009. The potential association between fruit intake and body weight – a review. *Obesity Reviews* 10(6), p. 639–647.
- Ahuja KDK et al 2006. Effects of chilli consumption on postprandial glucose, insulin, and energy metabolism. *The American journal of clinical nutrition* 84(1), p. 63–69.
- Aggarwal BB 2010. Targeting inflammation-induced obesity and metabolic diseases by curcumin and other nutraceuticals. *Annual review of nutrition* 30, p. 173–199.
- Srinivasan K 2005. Spices as influencers of body metabolism: an overview of three decades of research. *Food Research International* 38(1), p. 77–86.
- Yoshioka M et al 1995. Effects of red-pepper diet on the energy metabolism in men. *Journal of nutritional science and vitaminology* 41.6, p. 647.
- Higgins JA et al 2004. Resistant starch consumption promotes lipid oxidation. *Nutrition & Metabolism*, 1(8).
- Berti C et al 2005. Effect on appetite control of minor cereal and pseudocereal products. *British journal of nutrition* 94(05),

p. 850–858.

- Ledoux TA et al 2011. Relationship of fruit and vegetable intake with adiposity: a systematic review. *Obesity Reviews* 12(5), e143-e150.
- Higgins JA 2013. Resistant starch and energy balance: impact on weight loss and maintenance. *Critical Reviews in Food Science and Nutrition* (just accepted).
- Sartorelli DS et al 2008. High intake of fruits and vegetables predicts weight loss in Brazilian overweight adults. *Nutrition Research*, 28(4), p. 233–238.
- Vioque J et al 2008. Intake of fruits and vegetables in relation to 10 year weight gain among Spanish adults. *Obesity* 16.3, p. 664–670.
- Johnston KL et al 2010. Resistant starch improves insulin sensitivity in metabolic syndrome. *Diabetic Medicine* 27(4), p. 391–397.
- Fujioka K et al 2006. The effects of grapefruit on weight and insulin resistance: relationship to the metabolic syndrome. *Journal of medicinal food* 9(1), p. 49–54.
- Parikh S et al 2012. Adolescent fibre consumption is associated with visceral fat and inflammatory markers. *Journal of Clinical Endocrinology & Metabolism* 97(8), E1451–E1457.
- Shahidi, F., & Ambigaipalan, P. (2015). Phenolics and polyphenolics in foods, beverages and spices: Antioxidant activity and health effects – A review. *Journal of Functional Foods*, 18, p. 820-897.

Week 4

- EFSA 2012. Scientific opinion on the tolerable upper intake levels of eicosapentaenoic acid (EPA) and docosahexaenoic acid (DHA) and docosapentaenoic acid (DPA). EFSA Journal 10(7), p. 2815.
- Kris-Etherton PM et al 2002. Fish consumption, fish oil, omega-3 fatty acids, and cardiovascular disease. *Circulation* 106, p. 2747–2757.
- Gilsanz V et al 2010. Vitamin D status and its relation to muscle mass and muscle fat in young women. *Journal of Clinical Endocrinology & Metabolism* 95(4), p. 1595–1601.
- Summers LKM et al 2002. Substituting dietary saturated fat with polyunsaturated fat changes abdominal fat distribution and improves insulin sensitivity. *Diabetologia* 45.3, p. 369–377.
- Sergeev IN 2009. 1, 25-Dihydroxyvitamin D3 induces Ca2+mediated apoptosis in adipocytes via activation of calpain and caspase-12. *Biochemical and biophysical research communications* 384(1), p. 18–21.
- Rodríguez-Rodríguez E et al 2010. Associations between abdominal fat and body mass index on vitamin D status in a group of Spanish schoolchildren. *European journal of clinical nutrition* 64(5), p.461–467.
- Micha R et al 2009. Trans fatty acids: effects on metabolic syndrome, heart disease and diabetes. *Nature Reviews Endocrinology* 5(6), p. 335–344.
- He K et al 2009. Fish, long-chain omega-3 polyunsaturated fatty acids and prevention of cardiovascular disease – eat fish or take fish oil supplement? *Prog Cardiovasc Dis*. 52(2), p. 95–114.

- Thorsdottir I et al 2007. Randomised trial of weight-loss-diets for young adults varying in fish and fish oil content. *International journal of obesity* 31(10), p. 1560–1566.
- Parra D et al 2008. A diet rich in long-chain omega-3 fatty acids modulates satiety in overweight and obese volunteers during weight loss. *Appetite* 51.3, s. 676–680.
- Lorente-Cebrián S et al 2013. Role of omega-3 fatty acids in obesity, metabolic syndrome, and cardiovascular diseases: a review of the evidence. *Journal of Physiology and Biochemistry*, s. 1–19.
- Irmisch G et al 2007. Fatty acids and sleep in depressed inpatients. *Prostagland. Leukot. Essent. Fatty Acids*, 76, s. 1–7.
- Arias-Carrión O et al 2011. Biochemical modulation of the sleep–wake cycle: Endogenous sleep-inducing factors. *J. Neurosci. Res.* 89, s. 1143–1149. doi: 10.1002/jnr.22666
- Wallin A et al 2012. Fish Consumption, Dietary Long-Chain n-3 Fatty Acids, and Risk of Type 2 Diabetes Systematic review and meta-analysis of prospective studies. *Diabetes care* 35(4), s. 918–929.
- Norkost 3. En landsomfattende kostholdsundersøkelse blant menn og kvinner i Norge i alderen 18–70 år. IS-2000. Helsedirektoratet 2012.

Week 5

- Lohi S et al 2007. Increasing prevalence of coeliac disease over time. *Alimentary pharmacology & therapeutics* 26(9), p. 1217–1225.
- van den Broeck HC et al 2010. Presence of coeliac disease epitopes in modern and old hexaploid wheat varieties: wheat breeding may have contributed to increased prevalence of coeliac disease. *Theoretical and applied genetics* 121(8), p. 1527–1539.
- Teschemacher H 2003. Opioid receptor ligands derived from food proteins. *Current pharmaceutical design* 9(16), p. 1331–1344.
- Ifland JR et al 2009. Refined food addiction: a classic substance use disorder. *Medical hypotheses* 72(5), p. 518–526.
- Ludvigsson JF et al 2009. Small-intestinal histopathology and mortality risk in coeliac disease. *JAMA: the journal of the American Medical Association* 302(11), p. 1171–1178.
- Osborn O et al 2012. The cellular and signaling networks linking the immune system and metabolism in disease. *Nature medicine* 18(3), p. 363–374.
- Ouchi N et al 2011. Adipokines in inflammation and metabolic disease. *Nature Reviews Immunology* 11(2), p. 85–97.

Week 6

- Maslowski KM et al 2010. Diet, gut microbiota and immune responses. *Nature immunology* 12.1, p 5–9.
- Vrieze A et al 2012. Transfer of intestinal microbiota from lean donors increases insulin sensitivity in individuals with metabolic syndrome. *Gastroenterology* 143(4), p. 913–916.

- Ley RE 2010. Obesity and the human microbiome. *Current opinion in gastroenterology* 26(1), p. 5–11.
- Woodard GA et al 2009. Probiotics improve outcomes after Roux-en-Y gastric bypass surgery: a prospective randomised trial. *Journal of Gastrointestinal Surgery* 13(7), p.1198–1204.
- Le Chatelier E et al 2013. Richness of human gut microbiome correlates with metabolic markers. *Nature* 500(7464), p. 541–546.
- Cani PD et al 2007. Metabolic endotoxemia initiates obesity and insulin resistance. *Diabetes* 56(7), p. 1761–1772.
- Kalliomäki M et al 2008. Early differences in fecal microbiota composition in children may predict overweight. *The American journal of clinical nutrition* 87(3), p. 534–538.
- Lozupone CA et al 2012. Diversity, stability and resilience of the human gut microbiota. *Nature* 489(7415), p. 220–230.
- Foster JA 2013. Gut Feelings: Bacteria and the Brain. *Cerebrum: the Dana forum on brain science*. Vol. 2013. Dana Foundation.
- Kau AL et al 2011. Human nutrition, the gut microbiome and the immune system. *Nature* 474(7351), p. 327–336.

Week 7

- Anderson GH et al 2004. Dietary proteins in the regulation of food intake and body weight in humans. *The Journal of Nutrition* 134(4), p. 974–979.
- Guyenet SJ et al 2012. Regulation of food intake, energy balance, and body fat mass: implications for the pathogenesis and treatment of obesity. *Journal of Clinical Endocrinology & Metabolism* 97(3), p. 745–755.
- Due A et al 2004. Effect of normal-fat diets, either medium or high in protein, on body weight in overweight subjects: a randomised 1-year trial. *Int J Obes Relat Metab Disord* 28, p. 1283–90.
- Layman DK et al 2009. A moderate-protein diet produces sustained weight loss and long-term changes in body composition and blood lipids in obese adults. *J Nutr* 1395, p. 14–21.
- Halton TL et al 2004. The effects of high protein diets on thermogenesis, satiety and weight loss: a critical review. *Journal of the American College of Nutrition* 23(5), p. 373–385.
- Larsen TM et al 2010. Diets with high or low protein content and glycaemic index for weight-loss maintenance. *New England Journal of Medicine* 363(22), p. 2102–2113.
- Noakes M et al 2005. Effect of an energy-restricted, high-protein, low-fat diet relative to a conventional high-carbohydrate, low-fat diet on weight loss, body composition, nutritional status, and markers of cardiovascular health in obese women. *The American journal of clinical nutrition* 81(6), p. 1298–1306.
- Westerterp-Plantenga et al 2009. Dietary protein, weight loss, and weight maintenance. *Annual review of nutrition* 29, p. 21–41.

Week 8

- Oi-Kano Y et al (2008). Oleuropein, a phenolic compound in extra virgin olive oil, increases uncoupling protein 1 content in brown adipose tissue and enhances noradrenaline and adrenaline secretions in rats. *Journal of nutritional science and vitaminology* 54(5), p. 363–370.
- Paniagua et al 2007. Monounsaturated Fat-Rich Diet Prevents Central Body Fat Distribution and Decreases Postprandial Adiponectin Extression Induced by a Carbohydrate-rich Diet in Insulin-Resistant Subjects. *Diabetes Care* 30, p. 1717–1723.
- Assunção et al 2009. Effects of dietary coconut oil on the biochemical and anthropometric profiles of women presenting abdominal obesity. *Lipids* 44(7), p. 593–601.
- Clegg ME et al 2013. Combined medium-chain triglyceride and chilli feeding increases diet-induced thermogenesis in normal-weight humans. *European journal of nutrition* 52(6), p. 1579–1585.
- Han JR et al 2007. Effects of dietary medium-chain triglyceride on weight loss and insulin sensitivity in a group of moderately overweight free-living type 2 diabetic Chinese subjects. *Metabolism* 56(7), p. 985–991.
- Nagao K et al 2010. Medium-chain fatty acids: functional lipids for the prevention and treatment of the metabolic syndrome. *Pharmacological Research* 61(3), p. 208–212.

Week 9 (calcium)

- Abargouei, AS et al 2012. Effect of dairy consumption on weight and body composition in adults: a systematic review and meta-analysis of randomised controlled clinical trials. *International Journal of Obesity* 36(12), p. 1485–1493.
- Zemel MB et al 2005. Dairy augmentation of total and central fat loss in obese subjects. *International journal of obesity* 29(4), p. 391–397.
- Caron-Jobin M et al 2011. Elevated serum 25 (OH) D concentrations, vitamin D, and calcium intakes are associated with reduced adipocyte size in women. *Obesity* 19(7), p. 1335–1341.
- Cohen A et al 2013. Abdominal fat is associated with lower bone formation and inferior bone quality in healthy premenopausal women: a transiliac bone biopsy study. *Journal of Clinical Endocrinology & Metabolism* 98(6), p. 2562–2572.
- Bertone-Johnson ER et al 2005. Calcium and vitamin D intake and risk of incident premenstrual syndrome. *Archives of internal medicine* 165(11), p. 1246.
- Cribb PJ et al 2006. The effect of whey isolate and resistance training on strength, body composition, and plasma glutamine. *International journal of sport nutrition and exercise metabolism* 16(5), p. 494–509.

- Bendsen NT 2008. Effect of dairy calcium on fecal fat excretion: a randomised crossover trial. *International Journal of Obesity* 32(12), p. 1816–1824.
- Russell M et al 2010. Visceral fat is a negative predictor of bone density measures in obese adolescent girls. *Journal of Clinical Endocrinology & Metabolism* 95(3), p. 1247–1255.
- Faghih SH 2011. Comparison of the effects of cows' milk, fortified soy milk, and calcium supplement on weight and fat loss in premenopausal overweight and obese women. *Nutrition, Metabolism and Cardiovascular Diseases* 21(7), p. 499–503.
- Zhu et al 2013. Calcium plus vitamin D3 supplementation facilitated Fat loss in overweight and obese college students with very-low calcium consumption: a randomised controlled trial. *Nutr J* 12(1), p. 1–8.
- Chen M et al 2012. Effects of dairy intake on body weight and fat: a meta-analysis of randomised controlled trials. *The American Journal of Clinical Nutrition* 96(4), p. 735–747.
- Sanders TA 2012. Role of dairy foods in weight management. *The American Journal of Clinical Nutrition* 96(4), p. 687–688.
- Josse AR et al 2012. Diets higher in dairy foods and dietary protein support bone health during diet- and exercise-induced weight loss in overweight and obese premenopausal women. *Journal of Clinical Endocrinology & Metabolism* 97(1), p. 251–260.
- Van Loan M 2009. The role of dairy foods and dietary calcium in weight management. *Journal of the American College of Nutrition* 28(suppl), p.120–129.
- Ebeling, P. R., Daly, R. M., Kerr, D. A., & Kimlin, M. G. (2013). An evidence-informed strategy to prevent osteoporosis in Australia. *Med J Aust*, 198(2), p. 90-91.
- Totland, T. H., Melnæs, B. K., Lundberg Hallèn, N., Helland-Kigen, K. M., Lund Blix, N.A., Myhre, J. B., ... & Andersen, L. F. (2012). Norkost 3; A nationwide food consumption survey among men and women in Norway aged 18–70 years, 2010–11. Directorate of Health,Oslo. Available in Norwegian from: http://healthdirectorate. no/publikasjoner/norkost-3-en-landsomfattendekostholdsunde rsokelse-blant-menn-og-kvinner-i-norge-i-alderen-18-70-ar/ Publikasjoner/norkost-3-is-2000.pdf.

Week 9 (magnesium)

- He K et al 2006. Magnesium intake and incidence of metabolic syndrome among young adults. *Circulation*, 113(13), s. 1675–1682.
- Barbagallo M et al 2007. Magnesium metabolism in type 2 diabetes mellitus, metabolic syndrome and insulin resistance. *Archives of biochemistry and biophysics* 458(1), p. 40–47.
- Rayssiguier Y et al 2010. Magnesium deficiency and metabolic syndrome: stress and inflammation may reflect calcium activation. *Magnes Res* 23(2), p. 73–80.
- Bes-Rastrollo M 2009. Prospective study of nut consumption, long-term weight change, and obesity risk in women. *The American journal of clinical nutrition* 89(6), p. 1913–1919.
- Casas-Agustench P et al 2010. Nuts, inflammation and insulin resistance. *Asia Pacific journal of clinical nutrition* 19(1), p. 124.
- Hollis J et al 2007. Effect of chronic consumption of almonds on body weight in healthy humans. *British Journal of Nutrition* 98(3), p. 651–656.
- Mattes RD et al 2008. Impact of peanuts and tree nuts on body weight and healthy weight loss in adults. *The Journal of nutrition* 138(9), p.1741–1745.
- Nielsen FH et al 2010. Magnesium supplementation improves indicators of low magnesium status and inflammatory stress in adults older than 51 years with poor quality sleep. *Magnes Res* 23(4), p. 158–68.
- Rayssiguier Y 2006. High fructose consumption combined with low dietary magnesium intake may increase the incidence of the metabolic syndrome by inducing inflammation. *Magnes Res* 19(4), p. 237–43.

Week 10

- Yang HY et al 2012. Beneficial effects of catechin-rich green tea and inulin on the body composition of overweight adults. *British Journal of Nutrition* 107(05), p. 749–754.
- Tsuneki H, Ishizuka M, Terasawa M, Wu JB, Sasaoka Tog Kimura I. (2004). Effect of green tea on blood glucose levels and serum proteomic patterns in diabetic (db/db) mice and on glucose metabolism in healthy humans. *BMC pharmacology* 4(1), p. 18.
- Zuk PA et al 2002. Human adipose tissue is a source of multipotent stem cells. *Molecular biology of the cell* 13(12), p. 4279–4295.
- Jaenisch R et al 2003. Epigenetic regulation of gene expression: how the genome integrates intrinsic and environmental signals. *Nature genetics* 33, p. 245–254.
- Auvichayapat P et al 2008. Effectiveness of green tea on weight reduction in obese Thais: A randomised, controlled trial. *Physiology & behavior* 93(3), p. 486–491.
- Wu CH et al 2003. Relationship among habitual tea consumption, percent body fat, and body fat distribution. *Obesity research* 11(9), p. 1088–1095.
- Wolfram S et al 2006. Anti-obesity effects of green tea: From bedside to bench. *Molecular nutrition & food research* 50(2), p. 176–187.
- Thielecke F et al 2009. The potential role of green tea catechins in the prevention of the metabolic syndrome – a review. *Phytochemistry* 70(1), p. 11–24.

- Cooper R 2005. Medicinal benefits of green tea: Part I. Review of noncancer health benefits. *Journal of Alternative & Complementary Medicine* 11(3), p. 521–528.
- Wang JF et al 2000. A dose-response effect from chocolate consumption on plasma epicatechin and oxidative damage. *The Journal of nutrition* 130(8), s. 2115–2119.
- Matsui N et al 2005. Ingested cocoa can prevent high-fat diet-induced obesity by regulating the expression of genes for fatty acid metabolism. *Nutrition* 21(5), p. 594–601.
- Ferri C et al 2003. Mediterranean diet, cocoa and cardiovascular disease: a sweeter life, a longer life, or both? *J Hypertens* 21, p. 2231–2234.
- Hollenberg NK et al 1997. Aging, acculturation, salt intake and hypertension in the Kuna of Panama. *Hypertension* 29, p.171–176.
- Grassi D et al 2005. Short-term administration of dark chocolate is followed by a significant increase in insulin sensitivity and a decrease in blood pressure in healthy persons. *The American journal of clinical nutrition* 81(3), p. 611–614.
- Engler MB et al 2004. Flavonoid-rich dark chocolate improves endothelial function and increases plasma epicatechin concentrations in healthy adults. *Journal of the American College of Nutrition* 23(3), p. 197–204.
- Wan Y et al 2001. Effects of cocoa powder and dark chocolate on LDL oxidative susceptibility and prostaglandin concentrations in humans. *The American journal of clinical nutrition* 74(5), p. 596–602.
- Mao T et al 2000. Cocoa procyanidins and human cytokine transcription and secretion. *The Journal of nutrition* 130(8), p. 2093–2099.

Week 11

- Dennis EA et al 2010. Water Consumption Increases Weight Loss During a Hypocaloric Diet Intervention in Middle-aged and Older Adults. *Obesity* 18(2), p. 300–307.
- Keller U et al 2003. Effects of changes in hydration on protein, glucose and lipid metabolism in man: impact on health. *European Journal of Clinical Nutrition* 57, p. 69–74.
- Green E et al 2012. Altered processing of sweet taste in the brain of diet soda drinkers. *Physiol. Behav.* 107, p. 560–567.
- Adams GE et al 2008. Hydration effects on cognitive performance during military tasks in temperate and cold environments. *Physiology and Behavior* 93, p. 748–756.
- Armstrong LE et al 2012. Mild dehydration affects mood in healthy young women. *The Journal of nutrition* 142(2), p. 382–388.
- Ganio MS 2011. Mild dehydration impairs cognitive performance and mood of men. *British Journal of Nutrition* 106(10), p. 1535.

- Fowler SP et al 2008. Fueling the obesity epidemic? Artificially sweetened beverage use and long-term weight gain. *Obesity* 16(8), p. 1894–1900.
- Brown RJ et al 2009. Ingestion of diet soda before a glucose load augments glucagon-like peptide-1. *Diab care* 32(12), p. 2184–2186.
- Nettleton JA et al 2009. Diet soda intake and risk of incident metabolic syndrome and type 2 diabetes in the Multi-Ethnic Study of Atherosclerosis (MESA) *Diabetes Care* 32(4), p. 688–694.
- Stookey JD 2008. Drinking water is associated with weight loss in overweight dieting women independent of diet and activity. *Obesity* 16(11), p. 2481–2488.

Week 12

- Nedeltcheva AV et al 2009. Sleep curtailment is accompanied by increased intake of calories from snacks. *The American journal of clinical nutrition* 89(1), p. 126–133.
- Schmid SM et al 2008. A single night of sleep deprivation increases ghrelin levels and feelings of hunger in normal-weight healthy men. *Journal of sleep research* 17(3), p. 331–334.
- Conceição de Oliveira M et al 2003. Weight loss associated with a daily intake of three apples or three pears among overweight women. *Nutrition* 19(3), p. 253–256.
- Chong ZZ et al 2012. SIRT1: New avenues of discovery for disorders of oxidative stress. *Expert opinion on therapeutic targets* 16(2), p. 167–178.
- Lekli I et al 2010. Longevity nutrients resveratrol, wines and grapes. *Genes & nutrition* 5(1), p. 55–60.
- Ma H et al 2009. Expression of adiponectin and its receptors in livers of morbidly obese patients with non-alcoholic fatty liver disease. *J Gastroenterol Hepatol.* 24(2), p. 233–237.
- dos Santos Costa C et al 2011. Resveratrol upregulated SIRT1, FOXO1, and adiponectin and downregulated PPARγ1–3 mRNA expression in human visceral adipocytes. *Obesity surgery* 21(3), p. 356–361.
- Panchal SK et al 2012. Quercetin ameliorates cardiovascular, hepatic, and metabolic changes in diet-induced metabolic syndrome in rats. *The Journal of nutrition* 142(6), p. 1026–1032.
- Walle T 2011. Bioavailability of resveratrol. *Annals of the New York Academy of Sciences* 1215(1), p. 9–15.

INDEX